Health and Social Care Research Methods in Context

This is the first textbook to show how research using a range of qualitative and quantitative methods relates to improving health and social care practice.

The book shows how different research approaches are undertaken in practice and the challenges and strengths of different methodologies, thus facilitating students to make informed decisions when choosing which to use in their own research projects. The eleven chapters are each structured around different research methods and include:

- A brief overview of the research and research question
- Identification and overview of the research approach and associated methods selected to answer this question
- The sample and recruitment, including issues and challenges
- Ethical concerns
- Practical issues in undertaking the research approach
- Links between the research process and findings to health and social care values
- Links to the full research study
- Further reading

The book will be a required reading for all students of social work; social care; nursing; public health and health studies and particularly suitable for those on widening participation courses.

Liz Tilly is Founder and Director of Building Bridges Training, West Midlands, UK, and Senior Lecturer in Social Care, University of Wolverhampton, Wolverhampton, UK. Liz is strongly committed to the full inclusion of people with learning disabilities in all aspects of life and has had regular professional and social contact with people with learning disabilities for many decades.

Health and Social Care Research Methods in Context

Applying Research to Practice

Edited by Liz Tilly

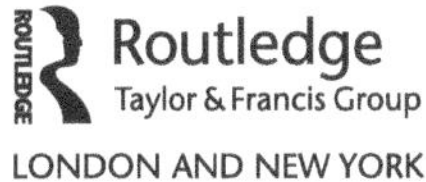

LONDON AND NEW YORK

First published 2022
by Routledge
2 Park Square, Milton Park, Abingdon, Oxon OX14 4RN

and by Routledge
605 Third Avenue, New York, NY 10158

Routledge is an imprint of the Taylor & Francis Group, an informa business

British Library Cataloguing-in-Publication Data
A catalogue record for this book is available from the British Library.

Library of Congress Cataloging-in-Publication Data
A catalog record has been requested for this book.

ISBN: 978-0-367-74422-9 (hbk)
ISBN: 978-0-367-74418-2 (pbk)
ISBN: 978-1-003-15772-4 (ebk)

DOI: 10.4324/9781003157724

Typeset in Helvetica
by Apex CoVantage, LLC

Contents

Contributors

Nahid Ahmad is an independent research consultant, UK. Nahid has previously held senior roles in both the academic sector and the private sector. She is a chartered psychologist with substantial expertise in evaluation and research. Nahid was formerly the deputy director of the Institute for Community Research and Development at the University of Wolverhampton and a member of the Violence Against Women and Girls Research Cluster (VAWGRC). Nahid's most recent work includes research for the Parental Alienation Study Group in which, along with co-researchers, she investigated the current service response to so-called parental alienation in the UK. She continues to be active in research in the field of parental alienation and has also delivered research and evaluation projects for NHS trusts and Clinical Commissioning Groups, local authorities, health charities and think tanks.

Andrew Beeput is CEO of the Bond Board, a not-for-profit specialist housing organisation in Bolton and Rochdale, UK.

Stephanie Brewster is Senior Lecturer at the University of Wolverhampton, UK. She teaches undergraduate and postgraduate students doing a variety of courses in Education, especially those studying special educational needs, disability and inclusion. She has an interest in inclusive teaching and learning and has worked extensively with students with additional needs in the higher education context. She is an active researcher in these fields and specialises in speech, language and communication needs amongst children and adults. Prior to this role she worked as a speech and language therapist with the National Health Service.

Katy Goldstraw is Senior Lecturer at Staffordshire University, UK, and a freelance researcher. Katy specialises in participatory and co-produced research.

Rachel Harrison is Senior Lecturer, University of Winchester, UK. Rachel's academic roles have included the leadership, design and delivery of degree programmes and consultancy to a range of statutory and charitable organisations and groups in the fields of health and social care. Rachel has a background of working with and for a range of young people and adults including disabled people and those who have intellectual and developmental disabilities. She previously managed residential services with and for people with dual diagnoses. Her PhD focused on how the lives and social networks of people with intellectual and developmental disabilities and their carers are impacted by austerity policies.

Jenni Jones is Associate Professor in Coaching and Mentoring at the University of Wolverhampton Business School, UK. She teaches undergraduate and postgraduate modules related to employability, diversity, coaching, mentoring, human resources, leadership and change. Her PhD research focused on mentoring and learning in the public sector, including healthcare and the police. Her research is predominantly qualitative and is focused on a broad range of topics related to learning, leadership, change, education and human resource development. She has presented at a number of conferences, published in a number of journals, including *Human Resource Development International*, *International Journal of Evidence Based Coaching and Mentoring* and *International Journal of Mentoring and Coaching* and co-edited a book for IGI Global.

Theresa Helen Kinnersley is Programme Director at NICE Centre for Movement Disorders, Birmingham, UK. Originally qualifying as a registered nurse, Theresa worked for the NHS within Neurology and Neurorehabilitation for 20 years before retraining and gaining a BA Hons in Conductive Education (with QCS) in 2005. The chapter entry is a 'snapshot' of her PhD which was completed in 2019. The research involved the use of a mixed-methods approach to explore and utilise perceptions of expertise in the construction of a Continuing Professional Development (CPD) tool.

Angela Morgan is Senior Researcher at the University of Wolverhampton, UK. Angela has worked as Senior Researcher for over 20 years. She is founder of the Violence Against Women and Girls Research Cluster at the university. Her research interests major in domestic abuse and the harm to children caused by family violence and parental alienation. She has supervised a number of doctoral students to successful completion in a variety of disciplines, and her methodological expertise sits in the qualitative paradigm and mixed-methods approaches to research. She has developed a portfolio of research on the subject of parental alienation and has worked with a number of international experts in this field.

Ani Murr is Senior Lecturer in Social Work at Wolverhampton University, UK. Ani is Practice Education Lead in the social work subject area, where she is responsible for the education and training of social work practice educators. Social work practice education is her key area of research interest.

Irtiza Qureshi is Research Fellow at the School of Medicine, University of Nottingham, UK. He specialises in researching issues around health, education and diversity. He has significant experience of working in the public sector, including developing policy in public health and children's services. He has been involved in various health services research including on issues around marginalised communities, mental health, COVID-19 and developing national networking capacity for Health Education England.

Liz Tilly is Founder and Director of Building Bridges Training, West Midlands, UK, and Senior Lecturer in Social Care, University of Wolverhampton, Wolverhampton, UK. Liz is strongly committed to the full inclusion of people with learning disabilities in all aspects of life and has had regular professional and social contact with people with learning disabilities for many decades. Building Bridges Training is a social enterprise of people with a learning disability. It provides training and does research focused on making a difference to people with a learning disability. She also founded and is involved in the registered charity Jigsaw Events, which provides people with a learning disability with social and leisure opportunities. Previously, she founded and for 20 years was Chief Executive of a voluntary organisation in the West Midlands, which provided a wide range of services and opportunities for people with learning disabilities. Prior to this, her career was in special education.

Colin Watt is Senior Lecturer in the School of Education and Social Work at Birmingham City University, UK. He is a registered social worker with extensive experience of operational child protection and safeguarding and strategic management in both statutory and voluntary sectors. Colin's research interests derive from his professional practice and include parenting and foster care, child protection and safeguarding and children's and young people's experiences of professional services.

1 Introduction

Liz Tilly

The reason for this book

During my years working as a senior lecturer at a widening participation higher education institution, I observed that both undergraduate and postgraduate students struggled with understanding research methodology, knowing which research methods best suited their research project and understanding how published research linked to practice. For many, research methods was a least enjoyed and even feared module, as it came with a whole new dictionary of terms and concepts. Many students choose a health and social care course after working in such roles in a paid or voluntary capacity and, prior to enrolling on their degree programme, they invariably have not encountered academic research, and many find it challenging to comprehend 'research', finding it the most difficult module on their programme.

While there are a range of books that provide a comprehensive guide to understanding qualitative and quantitative research methods, there are limited resources that explain how these methods are used in practice, particularly for health and social care students.

To address this issue, *Understanding Health and Social Care Research: Methods in Context* was conceived and developed.

Aims of the book

The aim is to help students following health and social care programmes to understand the relationship between social care issues, research methodology and how the findings from research studies can both improve and change practice. It will enable the reader to

DOI: 10.4324/9781003157724-1

relate social research methodology to social research studies done in the real world.

This book aims to also provide clear examples of different social research methodologies to help postgraduate students make an informed decision on the most appropriate research methods to use for their own research projects. It is intended to help students gain an understanding of how different research approaches are undertaken in practice – their strengths, limitations and the challenges involved.

Students are expected to demonstrate skill in being 'critical' and 'evaluative' but often these concepts can be difficult to grasp. Each chapter contains an appraisal of a research study completed by the author, including a reflective section, enabling the reader to appreciate the nature of critique.

The studies included in the book serve to highlight how societal changes and contemporary problems such as austerity, new populations in the UK, and increased awareness of inclusion and participation all require innovative research approaches in order to gain a deeper understanding of the key issues involved and greater appreciation of developments in the social world.

Knowledge transfer is also an increasingly important aspect of academic research. This book serves to illustrate the immense value and benefit to practice of innovative qualitative research studies in the field of health and social care. It also highlights the challenges of knowledge transfer and the importance of making the findings accessible to practitioners and policymakers in order to make a difference.

While a broad range of social research methods are covered in the chapters, providing a comprehensive guide to each method included, this book does not claim to provide coverage of all available social research methods.

Who the book is for

This textbook is for practice-based levels 3 to 6 students on social work, health/public health, nursing and social care programmes. The book will also be of value to practitioners who are planning to conduct health and social research projects in their workplace, as it gives an overview of the delivery of all aspects of a research project.

The book is designed to be accessible for students to pick up and read. The case studies are relevant to practice and their current future employment. It is written in plain English making it suitable for widening participation and international students – an increasing population in many university health and social care programmes.

The authors

Each chapter is written by an academic who has undertaken a recent research study as part of their own doctoral studies, as a postdoctoral project or as commissioned research. A link to their study, where available, is included in their chapter. A biography of each author and their contact details can be found in the preface of the book.

The book and chapter structure

Following this introductory chapter, the book contains ten chapters featuring a range of topics related to social care and different research methods used in health and social care research studies. Each chapter outlines how the studies were disseminated and their relevance to practice.

Each chapter follows the same structure to enable comparisons to be drawn by the reader:

- A brief overview of the research
- The research question(s)
- Identification of the research approach and the reason for the methods selected to answer the research questions (with references to research methodology texts)
- The challenges of selection and recruitment of the research sample

- The benefits of the approach taken and its application to the research topic
- Ethical concerns related to the study and how these were addressed
- Practical issues arising from the chosen research approach
- Links between the research process and the findings to health and social care values
- How the research project was disseminated
- The feasible impact on social care, nursing/public health practice, policy or education
- Lessons learnt and pointers for replicating the research study
- Links to the full research study
- A comparison summary of the strengths and weaknesses of the research method
- Further reading

Also contained within each chapter are one or two activities for students to help embed the learning from the chapter.

Ethical issues

As mentioned, each chapter covers the ethical issues relating to the specific research study and how these were addressed. These include how the researchers considered informed consent, anonymity, confidentiality, managing distress and data security.

These are specifically highlighted in each chapter as ethically sound research is of paramount importance when researching 'vulnerable' groups and the specific inclusion in each chapter enables students to understand the application of ethical considerations in both research and practice.

Social research methods explored

Some of the chapters use a participatory approach and describe research undertaken working alongside others who are in need of health and/or social care support. For example, the chapter on participatory research by Katy Goldstraw and Andrew Beeput focuses on people who attended an advice cafe, and my chapter on inclusive research concerns working with people with a learning disability as co-researchers.

Teaching experience has identified the fear and dread many health and social care students have about quantitative research using statistical analysis. Seeing how this research method is used in practice, as part of mixed methods studies in the chapters by Rachel Harrison, Irtiza Qureshi and Theresa Helen Kinnersley, will hopefully allay student's anxieties but also enable them to see how using this research approach can have an impact on practice.

Survey data and its analysis, and application to practice, is explained by Angela Morgan and Nahid Ahmad in their chapter. Colin Watt and Jenni Jones's chapters demonstrate how semi-structured interviews and thematic analysis can be used in research to explore contemporary issues. Ani Murr's chapter explains dialogical narrative analysis, and the chapter by Stephanie Brewster gives an account of an ethnographical study, demonstrating other qualitative methods in specific contexts.

The following table (Table 1.1) indicates, for each chapter, the research methodology and approach used and the focus group or topic of the research study.

Table 1.1 Health and Social Care Research Methods in Context
Edited book – chapter summary for Introduction Chapter **21.5.21**

	Author	*Research methodology used*	*Focus (group and/or topic)*
1.	Liz Tilly		
2.	Rachel Harrison	Mixed methods	People with a learning disability and austerity
3.	Liz Tilly	Inclusive research	People with a learning disability and social inclusion
4.	Angela Morgan and Nahid Ahmad	Online survey	Parental alienation

(*Continued*)

Table 1.1 (Continued)

	Author	*Research methodology used*	*Focus (group and/or topic)*
5.	Jenni Jones	Semi-structured interviews and focus groups	Workplace mentoring
6.	Colin Watt	Semi-structured interviews and thematic analysis	Care experienced young people and foster carers
7.	Katy Goldstraw and Andrew Beeput	Participatory research and creative methods	Vulnerable clients
8.	Ani Murr	Dialogical narrative analysis	Using stories to explore the experience of supporting and assessing social work students' practice learning
9.	Stephanie Brewster	Ethnography	Communication; people with severe learning disabilities
10.	Theresa Kinnersley	Mixed methods	Professional development applicable to person-centred professions
11.	Irtiza Qureshi	Mixed methods utilising intersectionalism	Ethnic minority men in the nursing profession

We hope you enjoy reading and using the book and would appreciate any feedback and comments.

Dr Liz Tilly
Building Bridges Training CIC
and
University of Wolverhampton

2 Using mixed methods in health and social care research

Rachel Harrison

This study used mixed methods to try to understand the effects of austerity (cuts to services, care and support) on people with a learning disability, parent carers and managers of services.

What is mixed methods research?

While there are many definitions of mixed methods research, in this chapter, mixed methods research refers to research which uses different types of approaches and measurement tools to find out different types of information about the people (participants) taking part in a research study. Research methods can be considered to be on a spectrum, with quantitative at one end and qualitative at the other. They are not in competition, but they do aim to find out different things.

Quantitative methods are concerned with finding out numbers, such as how many people in a particular area have tested positive for a virus, or whether a particular vaccine is more effective in one age group than another. Historically, quantitative measures were considered to be the most reliable way to undertake research and it is clear that collecting this kind of information is still vital in many types of research in health and social care. After much campaigning and critique of some quantitative research approaches by groups

DOI: 10.4324/9781003157724-2

of disabled people, women, and people from minority ethnic backgrounds, qualitative approaches and measures have begun to also be seen as an important way of undertaking research which promotes hearing a wider range of voices and experiences and sharing power (Robson, 2002).

Qualitative measures are usually used when we are trying to find out about why people do what they do or think what they think. This might help us understand *why* there are higher rates of homelessness in one area of the country than another, or how people in different age groups *experience* homelessness. Using both types of measures can then help researchers in health and social care to understand for example not only how many people are in a particular category (such as homeless people) but to also find out what being in that category means to them; to look behind the numbers to find out what the numbers might mean (Creswell and Plano Clark, 2011).

A piece of research using mixed methods might have two different types of measures: one set which asks quantitative questions and one set which uses qualitative questions. Or you might use one set of questions that includes both quantitative and qualitative questions. If you are asking both quantitative and qualitative questions, you are undertaking mixed methods research (Kumar, 2018, pp. 14–16). You might use questionnaires for both quantitative and qualitative types of questions, or interviews for both, or you might use different ways of asking questions for each type, like an online questionnaire for quantitative questions (how many, when, where questions) and an interview for qualitative questions (why, how does this happen, what is your experience questions).

Undertaking research and having the ability to think about what questions you need to ask in order to get the information you need has clear links to employability skills. You will need organisational, time management and critical thinking skills in order to develop and create your own piece of research. Undertaking your first research project gives you the opportunity to hone these skills, which you can then use in your workplace.

Research question: What is the impact of care status on the quality of life and social networks of people with a learning disability?

Activity 1

Using more than one method can provide opportunities for researchers to gain a wider range of different types of information. The key consideration is: what is it you want to find out in your research project? When you know this, you can then begin to think about the best ways to go about trying to gain the information you need to answer your research question. What are you interested in finding out about? Make a list of your interests starting with broad ideas and moving to being as specific as possible.

Benefits and drawbacks of mixed methods research

Advantages

- Capturing and using information and experiences from diverse people in diverse ways
- Insights into participants' experiences that might be missed if just one form of research approach or tool is used
- Can double-check responses, asking questions in different ways and in different formats
- An added level of nuance and understanding in your research

Disadvantages

- The more methods we use, the harder it can be to make sense of different data given in different ways.
- Additional time may mean additional inconvenience for participants.

How to create mixed methods

It can be useful to ask yourself four key questions before you start any research project. These are:

- What is my main research question?
- What is/are my aim(s) (what am I trying to achieve with this research project)?
- What are my objectives (smaller questions which added together will answer my main question)?
- What are the best methods to use to answer each of my objectives, my aims and question?

In the case study example given later, you will be able to see how a real mixed methods research project was designed using these four key questions.

It is useful to consider what you want to find out about and why. From this you can build your research objectives, aim and main research question. You can then begin to consider how you might go about gathering the information you will need to answer your question. In your first research project, such as a dissertation, keeping your methods simple, short and clear is a good way to try to ensure your methods are appropriate for the task.

Making sure your methods enhance and add depth to your research question is important; they should form a coherent 'suite' or 'family' of methods which has a core aim which is clear to you and your participants. Each method you use should answer a different aspect of your research question. For example, you may choose to have three objectives in your research, one of which you hope to illuminate with a quantitative measure, one with a qualitative measure and one which draws on your responses from both measures combined.

Your mixed methods will need to be appropriate to your target group of participants. You should ask yourself:

- Will information and questionnaires need to be in easy-read language or have pictures and symbols?

- If you want to use a scale (strongly agree to strongly disagree for example) what scale will you use and how many measures will you have within it?
- If self-completion questionnaires are part of your set of methods, how will you get them to participants and how will they be returned?
- If you intend to interview participants yourself, or hold focus groups, will you audio/video record and/or take notes?
- Where will interviews take place?
- Who will transcribe any recordings?
- You will need to consider your own safety and comfort as well as that of your participant. If you intend to use observation, interviews or focus groups, what will you do about members of the public or families who visit the place of observation but may not be part of your research study?
- Where will you store all the data you gain?
- How will you ensure you are behaving ethically – including having permission from an ethics panel to undertake research?
- Who will support you in your research?

When considering these and the many other questions which will arise before, during and after your research project has taken place, it is useful to plan effectively and do a 'trial-run' first. This gives you the opportunity to try out your mixed methods and measures on friends, family or colleagues to get their feedback on whether they could make sense of your methods and whether you could make sense of their responses.

When you have refined your measures and methods, it is good practice to undertake a 'pilot study' with participants who will not form part of your main study. This gives you the opportunity to check not only whether your methods are appropriate but also whether your research question, aims and your mixed methods approach are meaningful to participants who are similar to those you intend to include in your research (Gomm, 2008). A question that is very clear and obvious to you may make no sense to a participant in your study, which may annoy participants or may mean you get a range of answers which do not relate to the question as you meant it.

The case study

The main research question was: What is the impact of care status on the quality of life and social networks of people with a learning disability? The aim was to gather evidence to be able to find out whether there was a link between participants' care and their quality of life and social networks. Social networks can contain a range of people, including partners, family, friends, acquaintances, professionals and neighbours. The research took place in England, with participants in the south of England and in the north east of England.

In this PhD study 56 people with a learning disability were interviewed using a range of questionnaires which used both qualitative and quantitative questions. Their responses were put into one of four categories which described what had happened with their care and support over the last ten years. Participants in the study either:

had no changes to their care and support;

or

had gained more care;

or

had lost some or all of their care;

or

the amount of care they had had stayed the same, but the type or place of care had changed.

Ten parent carers and nine managers of care services (one of whom was a government worker) were also separately interviewed and asked about their experiences of cuts to care.

To answer the aim and the main research question there were four objectives for this research project, which were:

1. Undertake a systematic literature review and synthesis to inform the study.
2. Using a range of quantitative measures, assess, analyse and report the care status, quality of life and social networks of 56 adults with a learning disability across two areas of the country over the last ten years.

3. Using qualitative, semi-structured interviews analyse and report the possible effects of changes to care status as experienced by parent carers.
4. Using qualitative, semi-structured interviews analyse and report the possible effects of changes to care status as experienced by managers of services for adults with a learning disability.

This research was important because understanding more about possible links between people's care, their social networks and their quality of life can help policymakers to understand the effects of their decisions; and ignoring these aspects of our lives comes at a human and financial cost. Social networks can combat loneliness (Callus, 2017), which can have a detrimental effect on health and well-being. This kind of research is particularly important for people in health and social care settings, as austerity policies since 2006 have reduced the eligibility for a wide range of personal and community care services for people with learning disability (Harrison, 2019; Malli et al., 2018).

The literature review was used to find out what information had been previously published on this topic (Harrison et al., 2021). The literature was analysed to find the key themes from research that had already been undertaken (Braun and Clarke, 2006). Reviewing the literature is important so that you can base your research questions in solid evidence and do not spend time and effort repeating a study that has already been carried out, without knowing about it.

To answer the second objective, five quantitative measures were used. These were:

- The Austerity Measure (created for the project by Professor Glynis Murphy)
- The Client Service Receipt Inventory for BLESS-A (CSRI) (Chisholm et al., 2000)
- The Glasgow Anxiety Scale for People with Learning Disability (GAS-ID, Mindham and Espie, 2003)
- The adapted Rosenberg Self-Esteem Measure (Dagnan and Sandhu, 1999)
- The Personal Outcomes Scale for Adults (POS) (van Loon, 2014)

The Social Network and Employability Scale (SONES) (Murphy, Gardner and Freeman, 2017) incorporating the Social Network Guide (see Forrester-Jones and Broadhurst, 2007) was also used. This is a mixed methods questionnaire as it has both quantitative questions (such as how many friends do you see each week?) and qualitative questions (such as who is your best friend and why?).

These measures were used to gather information on the details of people's lives which could then be used to better understand the nature of cuts to care for people with a learning disability.

To answer the third and fourth objectives, ten parent carers and nine managers of services were separately audio-recorded in semi-structured interviews asking them about their experiences of austerity and cuts to care, support or services. Mangers of services were asked general qualitative questions about the effects of cuts on the people they supported and on their services. Parent carers were asked general qualitative questions about the effects of cuts on themselves and on their families, including on social networks. All participants were encouraged to talk about topics which were important to them, and broad interview questions were used as a guide, such as, 'Can you tell me about any effects of austerity or cuts to services?'.

Two methods of analysis were used to better understand the data that was gathered. SPSS is a statistical software package which researchers can use to enter their quantitative data and undertake different tests on that data to find out if there are any links between participants' answers to different questions. This was used for the information that people with a learning disability gave in their interviews. For the semi-structured interviews with parent carers and with managers Interpretative Phenomenological Analysis (IPA) was used. IPA uses 'phenomenology' to consider subjective experience, often of relationships. This means IPA focuses on the experience of a small number of participants and what meanings can be made from the experiences they share (Smith, Flowers and Larkin, 2012).

Sample and recruitment

Difficulties arose in sampling as several local authorities chose not to take part. Without this and without access to a full and complete national database of people with a learning disability, it was difficult to include a sample of people who represented each care status group equally, or to include in the sample people from a range of ethnicities or a range of sexual preferences for example. Only one homosexual married couple were found, which may represent a wider issue around marriage rights for people with a learning disability.

National and local charities and groups were contacted by email and groups of disabled people, families and organisations were visited in a call to recruit people with a learning disability to take part in a wider project regarding austerity and its effects on people within this group and their families. This meant people who took part were 'self-selecting': they took part because they had an agenda of their own. Despite this, almost equal numbers of people who had lost care and whose care had stayed the same took part.

What did we have to think about?

This project and the amount of work involved took significant resources in terms of time, effort and funding. Travelling around the country to interview people took time and effort and cost money, all of which needs to be factored into your research. As with much research, all responses relied on participants' memories, their understanding of the questions, researcher-bias and power differentials between participant and researcher (Charmaz, 2014). While self-completed questionnaires would have been more cost- and time-efficient, there was an opportunity for misunderstanding of questions (Grix, 2010) and lack of opportunity to share the full experiences of participants. People with a learning disability would most likely have needed support to complete the questionnaires online; many participants had no internet access and/or had high levels of learning impairment. Lack of access to possible participants reduces the amount of people who can be involved and raises questions about the answers given, especially in a sensitive topic such as care. Focus groups too would have been more time-efficient and may have offered opportunities for participants to share experiences, for people with learning disability, parent carers and for managers. However, they are also open to the pressures of group dynamics, which may have led to participants' experiences being expressed in ways they would not ordinarily choose (Foster-Turner, 2009) or not expressed at all. Requiring participants to attend a focus group at a specific time and place may also exclude people who need time, support and access to transport in order to attend meetings.

Ethical issues

Researchers must work ethically, transparently and with explicit consent as a fundamental way to empower and understand participants as human beings influenced by their socio-historical context (Groundwater-Smith, 2009; Lincoln and Guba, 1985) and reflexively tackle the power imbalances inherent in the research process. Coercion and acquiescence are key issues regularly raised as part of the discussion around power and research (Cameron and Murphy, 2007); the position of the researcher must therefore be fully agreed, clarified and critiqued (Walmsley, 2004); hence the use of appropriate easy-read and picture information and support. The burden was minimised by offering breaks and ensuring interviews were timed to suit participants. Independent help and advice were available to all participants through an agreement between the university funding this PhD research and a national support charity for people with a learning disability and their families.

Making sure you have support for yourself before any ethical dilemmas or distressing situations arise is very important. Participants did report abusive situations in this PhD study, so you should plan to have clear reporting measures in place, to be clear yourself and with participants at the start that if you uncover any issues you may have to report those to your supervisor, and that may include reporting to the police and social services. People can then decide to participate or not and can make informed decisions about their responses, with everyone being clear about how any issues of concern will be handled.

Research outcomes: lessons learnt

The strengths of the method employed were that people with a learning disability, parent carers and managers could share information about their lives and about their experiences in a range of different ways. Enabling participants to share their experiences about what was important to them meant a holistic approach could flourish, where many voices were heard and respected and contributed to our understanding of how different people were experiencing cuts to services, care and support.

The main challenge for this study lay in accessing large numbers of people with a learning disability. Building trust with charities who could give access was essential, worthwhile, productive and time-consuming. Many participants were busy; and others found answering a large number of questions could be quite tiring. Nevertheless, the ways in which cuts could be experienced provided insights which may otherwise have been missed, from voices that are often unheard.

This research added considerably to health and social care values as it enabled a range of people who are often left out of the research process to be included and share issues which were important to them. This was done in ways that were respectful and empowering including proactively seeking out the people who are often excluded from mainstream discussions and policy and ensuring those people have the opportunity to share their voices and take part in research about policies which affect them, respecting their lives and experiences.

Key findings of this research project

- Cuts to care had negatively impacted many people with a learning disability in this study in terms of their health, care, support, services and welfare benefits. Their social networks and quality of life had been affected.

- Providers raised concerns about the effects of cuts on the lives of people with a learning disability. This included their health, well-being, activities, social networks and quality of life.
- Parents, especially older parents, were finding many aspects of their lives harder as services were cut.

What did we do with our learning?

Initial indications from the research were presented at International Association for the Scientific Study of Learning Disability conferences. The overarching research project (of which this PhD project was a part) was disseminated on the website of the National Institute of Health Research School for Social Care Research; on the Tizard Centre, University of Kent website; on the University of Winchester website and in this chapter. The literature review part of this study was published in March 2021 in the *Journal of Applied Research in Intellectual Disabilities*. Further academic articles are planned.

Implications for policy: understanding the effects of policies on the lives of people affected by those policies is essential in order that policies can be effective and be reviewed using evidence. Providing this evidence about the effects of austerity on the lives of people with learning disability, parent carers and managers of services can therefore positively influence current policy review and future policymaking.

Implications for practice: understanding the ways in which people with a learning disability, families and managers experience the effects of cuts to their care, services and benefits can provide evidence for people in these groups to use when advocating for their needs. It can also provide a basis for managers when planning services to best meet people's needs and for local authorities to better understand the effects of the financial cuts they make.

On reflection if you were to do this research study again, what would you do differently?

When interviewing people with learning disability quantitatively, many people gave more qualitative information than was required. Next time, having semi-structured interviews with people with a learning disability using a recording device to capture their additional information would be helpful, so that their actual words could be used with more academic weight and rigour, if they felt that was appropriate for them.

Activity 2

Test your knowledge and understanding of how to design a mixed methods study in health and social care research by creating a list of questions you could ask to find out more about your research topic. Are these questions quantitative, or qualitative, or both?

Link to the full research study

NIHR SSCR. (2020). *Becoming less eligible? Learning disability services in the age of austerity*, Research Findings 100. London: NIHR School for Social Care Research. [online] Available at: www.sscr.nihr.ac.uk/wp-content/uploads/SSCR-research-findings_RF100.pdf [Accessed 1 Feb. 2021].

Further reading

Creswell, J.W. and Clark, V.L.P. (2017). *Designing and conducting mixed methods research.* Thousand Oaks, CA: Sage.

The Money, Friends and Making Ends Meet Research Group c/o Liz Tilly. (2012). Having friends – they help you when you are stuck from money, friends and making ends meet research group. *British Journal of Learning Disabilities*, 40(2), pp. 128–133. doi: org/10.1111/j.1468-3156.2012.00739.x.

References

Braun, V. and Clarke, V. (2006). Using thematic analysis in psychology. *Qualitative Research in Psychology*, 3, pp. 77–101. [online] Available at: https://doi.org/10.1191/1478088706qp063oa [Accessed 1 Feb. 2021].

Callus, A.M. (2017). 'Being friends means helping each other, making coffee for each other': Reciprocity in the friendships of people with learning disability. *Disability and Society*, 32(1), pp. 1–16. [online] Available at: https://doi.org/10.1080/09687599.2016.1267610 [Accessed 1 Feb. 2021].

Cameron, L. and Murphy, J. (2007). Obtaining consent to participate in research: The issues involved in including people with a range of learning and communication disability. *British Journal of Learning Disability*, 35(2), pp. 113–120. [online] Available at: https://doi.org/10.1111/j.1468-3156.2006.00404.x [Accessed 1 Feb. 2021].

Charmaz, K. (2014). *Constructing grounded theory*, 2nd ed. London: Sage.

Chisholm, D., Knapp, M.R.J., Knudsen, H.C., Amaddeo, F., Gaite, L.U.I.S., Van Wijngaarden, B.O.B. and EPSILON Study Group. (2000). Client socio-demographic and service receipt inventory – European version: Development of an instrument for international research: EPSILON study 5. *The British Journal of Psychiatry*, 177(S39), pp. 28–33. [online] Available at: https://doi.org/10.1192/bjp.177.39.s28 [Accessed 1 Feb. 2021].

Creswell, J.W. and Plano Clark, V.L. (2011). *Designing and conducting mixed methods research*, 2nd ed. Thousand Oaks, CA: Sage.

Dagnan, D. and Sandhu, S. (1999). Social comparison, self-esteem and depression in people with learning disability. *Journal of Learning Disability Research*, 43(5), pp. 372–379. [online] Available at: https://doi: org/10.1046/j.1365-2788.1999.043005372.x.

Forrester-Jones, R.V.E. and Broadhurst, S. (2007). *Autism and loss*. London: Jessica Kingsley Publishers.

Foster-Turner, J. (2009). Focus groups. In: J. Neale, ed., *Research methods for health and social care*. Basingstoke: Palgrave Macmillan, pp. 211–223.

Gomm, R. (2008). *Social research methodology: A critical introduction*. Basingstoke: Palgrave Macmillan.

Grix, J. (2010). *The foundations of research*, 2nd ed. Basingstoke: Palgrave Macmillan.

Groundwater-Smith, S. (2009). Action research. *Educational Action Research*, 17(3), pp. 479–481. [online] Available at: https://doi.org/10.1080/09650790903088037 [Accessed 1 Feb. 2021].

Harrison, R.A. (2019). Commentary on "Afraid to leave the house: Issues leading to social exclusion and loneliness for people with a learning disability". *Tizard Learning Disability Review*, 24(4), pp. 176–179. [online] Available at: https://doi.org/10.1108/TLDR-08-2019-0026 [Accessed 1 Feb. 2021].

Harrison, R.A., Bradshaw, J., Forrester-Jones, R., McCarthy, M. and Smith, S. (2021). Social networks and people with intellectual disabilities: A systematic review. *Journal of Applied Research in Intellect Disabilities*. https://doi.org/10.1111/jar.12878 [Accessed 26 Apr. 2021].

Kumar, R. (2018). *Research methodology: A step-by-step guide for beginners*. Thousand Oaks, CA: Sage.

Lincoln, Y.S. and Guba, E.G. (1985). *Naturalistic inquiry*. London: Sage.

Malli, M.A., Sams, L., Forrester-Jones, R., Murphy, G. and Henwood, M. (2018). Austerity and the lives of people with learning disability. A thematic synthesis of current literature. *Disability and Society*, 33(9), pp. 1412–1435. [online] Available at: https://doi.org/10.1080/09687599.2018.1497950 [Accessed 1 Feb. 2021].

Mindham, J. and Espie, C.A. (2003). Glasgow anxiety scale for people with an learning disability (GAS-ID): Development and psychometric properties of a new measure for use with people with mild learning disability. *Journal of Learning Disability Research*, 47(1), pp. 22–30. [online] Available at: https://doi.org/10.1046/j.1365-2788.2003.00457.x [Accessed 1 Feb. 2021].

Murphy, G.H., Gardner, J. and Freeman, M.J. (2017). Screening prisoners for learning disability in three English prisons. *Journal of Applied Research in Learning Disability*, 30(1), pp. 198–204. [online] Available at: https://doi.org/10.1111/jar.12224 [Accessed 1 Feb. 2021].

Robson, C. (2002). *Real world research: A resource for social scientists and practitioner-researchers*. Oxford: Wiley-Blackwell.

Smith, J.A., Flowers, P. and Larkin, M. (2012). *Interpretative phenomenological analysis: Theory, method and research*. London: Sage.

van Loon, J. (2014). Personal outcomes scale. In: A.C. Michalos, ed., *Encyclopedia of quality of life and well-being research*. Dordrecht: Springer, pp. 4744–4747.

Walmsley, J. (2004). Inclusive learning disability research: The (nondisabled) researcher's role. *British Journal of Learning Disability*, 32(2), pp. 65–71. [online] Available at: https://doi.org/10.1111/j.1468-3156.2004.00281.x [Accessed 1 Feb. 2021].

3 Inclusive research – as a strategy for improving inclusive communities

Liz Tilly

Introduction

This chapter outlines the benefits and challenges of doing research with co-researchers with a learning disability, an approach termed 'inclusive research' (Walmsley and Johnson, 2003). It will first outline the main features of inclusive research methodology, then describe a recent research project undertaken by an inclusive research group.

Research about people with disabilities has traditionally been done by non-disabled people, by relatively powerful experts on relatively powerless 'subjects', and therefore on an unequal basis (Ward and Flynn, 1994). Decades ago, people with a learning disability were not asked their opinions and choices, instead their parents or staff were asked to speak for them. However, from the late 1960s, changes in attitude meant that people with a learning disability started to be consulted for their personal views, and the path towards genuine participation commenced (Walmsley, 2001).

Although research about people with a learning disability has been slow to involve them in the process at any level (Kiernan, 1999), they are increasingly taking a more active role. There has been a development from accepting that people with learning disabilities have opinions and the right to express them, and that they are the best informants concerning their experiences (Chappell, 2000), towards an understanding that speaking up about one's

DOI: 10.4324/9781003157724-3

experiences is a fundamental human right (United Nations, 2007). As a result, research conducted in collaboration with people with learning disabilities is taking an increasingly prominent place in current literature on learning disability-related issues (Walmsley, 2001; Nind, 2014).

The emergence of the social model of disability from the late 1970s identified the disabling factor to be the social barriers experienced, as opposed to a person's impairments (Barnes and Mercer, 2004). This social movement has enabled the development of an approach to research where people with disabilities are equal partners. Typically, disability research tends to consider the experience of disability or the structural barriers, which can be considered to be oppositional. Emancipatory research, where people with impairments are central to both the process and analysis, can be challenging for those with a learning disability to achieve without support. There are, however, calls for all research concerning people with learning disabilities to be emancipatory and to lead to real social change (Watson, 2004; Oliver, 1992). Inclusive research is grounded in these values and is an approach where support is an integral feature, yet provided without undermining the ownership of the research project (Walmsley, Strnadová and Johnson, 2018).

Inclusive research is also known by other names: co-research, collaborative, user-led, partnership and participatory research (Nind, 2014). There is no scope here to explain the history and nuances between these terms and approaches. For the purpose of this chapter, inclusive research is understood to be where people with a learning disability identify the research topic, take a lead role in all aspects of the research process (with support), including deciding the research topic, methodology, analysis and dissemination, which means they are far more than just data informants (Walmsley and Johnson, 2003; Walmsley, Strnadová and Johnson, 2018; Nind, 2017). It acknowledges that people with a learning disability are best placed to identify the social barriers they experience and the societal changes that should be made. It gives voice not only to their experience but also their own way of communicating this (Herron, Priest and Read, 2015).

The Building Bridges Research Group

Building Bridges is a social enterprise which was established to co-deliver training about learning disability to paid workers and deliver short courses for people with a learning disability. The research group started in 2010 when a short-term project was established to enable a group of people with a learning disability to 'research their own lives' using focus groups and creative activities. They completed the project by producing a report of their findings (Money Friends and Making Ends Meet Research Group, 2011).

The members greatly valued the opportunity to meet regularly and tell their stories, with the status of being researchers. Over ten years later, the group is still meeting regularly to research issues affecting them in their social networks (Building Bridges Research Group, 2014; Building Bridges Research Group, 2016). They have also written, or contributed to, a number of peer-reviewed journal articles (Mooney, Rafique and Tilly, 2019; Tilly, 2019a, 2013a, 2013b, 2014, 2016; Tilly and Building Bridges Research Group, 2015). Subjects have included housing, welfare benefits, coping with independent living, health and managing money and enabling professionals and academics to better comprehend their challenges in daily living. The group has seen changes in membership over the years, but it averages eight members. The members mainly live independently, and none have any support from learning disability services. It must be noted however that this group, whilst the largest in the learning disability population, is not representative of all people with a learning disability, namely those with severe and profound learning disability.

Barriers to community involvement

The following describes a recent inclusive research project delivered by the group. When carrying out an inclusive research project, the research topic and research question arise completely or partially from the researchers with a learning disability and their lived experience. My role as the group facilitator involved drawing together the group's discussions about the social barriers they experienced to form the research question. It is important that researchers with a learning disability understand the research question and that it is within their abilities, with support, to find answers to it.

Research aim

This research project explored the barriers that prevent people with a learning disability from being more involved with local people in community venues and activities and from building more friendships. The group were then supported to consider how those barriers could be challenged and changed.

Ethics and consent

Informed consent is difficult for people with a learning disability, despite the provision of accessible information sheets and consent forms. The researchers may not fully understand what they are consenting to or appreciate the reach of the dissemination, especially if it is outside their experience. An important ethical consideration is that people with a learning disability often have unfulfilled lives and therefore may agree to participate to fill otherwise unoccupied time. This creates a dilemma when recruiting research participants but is particularly problematic when recruiting co-researchers, where the role is even more complex.

The researchers in this project signed an easy read consent form at the beginning of the research project and agreed to ground rules at the beginning of each meeting. For example, it was agreed that 'what's said in the room stays in the room'. We also used traffic-light cards to manage any situations where people broke the ground rules. Thus red, yellow and green cards were used to interrupt or pause the meeting if someone was unhappy about something. We agreed not to talk about personal feelings about being lonely in this setting, and if anyone felt sad they didn't have to stay in the discussion and would get support.

Data collection

The researchers participated in four focus groups to identify some of the specific barriers that prevented them from having community inclusion and the opportunity to develop friends. The discussions were recorded on a digital recorder and were transcribed by a third party. I then read through the notes and summarised them into a long list of all the key thoughts and issues we had talked about. One of the group members produced large pictorial cards for each of the issues.

These cards were used to undertake a thematic analysis through a group sorting exercise. We put all the picture cards on the table and worked together to put the cards into groups of similar issues. We then gave these groups names such as 'family', 'money' or 'anxiety'. These themes then enabled the group to discuss suggestions for ways to overcome these barriers and so increase access to community activities and expand their social networks. These overarching themes are discussed here in the context of the following wider literature.

Key findings

Travel, community safety and anxiety

The inclusive research project (Mooney, Rafique and Tilly, 2019) found that while people did not report personal experiences of harassment or abuse, they feared going out alone, especially at night. These fears were magnified by hearing of increased reports of gun and knife crime. They also reported lack of confidence in using public transport, especially where more than one journey had to be made, and fear of getting lost in strange places, which was identified as a barrier to going to community places. A further restriction, particularly in the winter months, was an aversion to travelling when it was dark outside.

Those who had a smartphone and used map and travel apps found them helpful, as they could locate where they were and find the nearest bus stops and when buses were due. The apps were also used on bus journeys to inform the passenger when to alight.

However, most people only had simple pay-as-you-go phones and were not able to use this technology.

With regard to perceived safety, the group stated that they would like there to be more 'Safe Places' in the community, identified by stickers on their doors and windows. This would enable people to know they could find a source of help and support when out in the community, should they experience any problems.

Choice and control

In the inclusive research project, some people reported restrictions over their choices and control within family relationships. These were due to both overprotectiveness and the issue of control over how much disability welfare benefit could be spent on social and leisure activities. This often led to frustration and disappointment when it resulted in not being able to join in activities with friends, such as going for a meal.

Access to information and digital exclusion

In the inclusive research project, the group said they wanted more 'easy read' information about what was available locally and suggested this could usefully be located in health settings, bus and train stations and places of worship. An easy read document contains minimal text, using simple words and short sentences. Pictures and photographs enable the reader to understand the content. It is also presented in a simple format and uses larger font (Department of Health, 2010; Inclusion Europe, n/k). They felt that local information should also include travel advice and maps to aid navigation.

Their findings and suggestions made only minimal references to technology and digital information; few had access to personal devices or broadband, so not all were aware of how technology and the internet could be helpful in furthering community inclusion. Their lack of awareness of this resource highlighted that this group of people continue to experience digital exclusion. Many people with learning disabilities have limited internet access and sometimes also limited skills to develop these connections. Furthermore, they frequently do not have smart devices which heightens the digital exclusion (Department for Communities and Local Government, 2008; Chadwick, Wesson and Fullwood, 2013).

How was this research project disseminated?

We wrote an article as an inclusive research piece, and I then produced a further article reflecting on the findings at a deeper level. We delivered presentations on this research project at two conferences and used it to inform presentations we made to social work students on university courses (Mooney, Rafique and Tilly, 2019; Tilly, 2019a, 2019b).

Activity 1

Think about some of the practical challenges for people with a learning disability to attend an academic conference and think of some creative ways to overcome these barriers.

Advantages and disadvantages of inclusive research

Advantages	*Disadvantages*
➢ An inclusive research approach gives a direct voice to marginalised groups and provides rich evidence of their lived experience. ➢ The process itself is empowering and enables rights to be upheld. ➢ Participation in a research group can bring immense personal benefits. Membership of the group provides a range of functions such as friendship, fun, peer support and an opportunity to identify and resolve issues and social barriers. ➢ Other outcomes include increased confidence and assertiveness among the members and heightened awareness of their rights.	➢ The process can take a lot longer as it requires much more preparation time to enable the researchers to be involved. ➢ It can be challenging to get people with a learning disability fully involved with in-depth analysis and the literature review – these aspects of the research process need much more support. ➢ Typically, the findings of inclusive research relate to a local group or area and there are limits to how far the findings can be generalised. ➢ There can be additional costs in delivering an inclusive research project, e.g. running group meetings.

(*Continued*)

(Continued)

Advantages	*Disadvantages*
➢ It affords people with a learning disability the status of experts, with respect and acknowledgement as researchers and authors. ➢ It has a huge impact on the professionals and students who hear their first-hand accounts.	➢ Costs for a small group to travel to conferences can be excessive, as opposed to a single researcher attending, as in traditional research. ➢ It is difficult for people with a severe or profound learning disability to participate due to the conceptual skills it requires.

Reflections on using inclusive research

Validity and equality

Inclusive research requires a strong rapport between all group members. A non-disabled researcher cannot suddenly decide to work inclusively and launch into it. It needs an environment of trust and for relationships to be nurtured and built up over time. There also needs to be consideration of roles and equality of power in the decision-making. While the non-disabled researcher may have different roles in the research project, such as managing budgets, leading on accountability and reporting to funders, there must be equality in the research process. The academic researcher may be more articulate, but the co-researchers are the ones with the lived experience and unique insight into both the challenges and solutions. It is this shared partnership that adds value to inclusive research (Nind, 2017).

It is important that co-researchers are not involved just for 'lip service' but in a genuine and meaningful way, and that participatory research is not wrongly labelled as inclusive. Inclusive research is extremely time-consuming, for example preparing easy read information or taking time to explain, remind and assure. But making reasonable adjustments can enable greater inclusion and therefore generate more pertinent research findings (Northway, Howarth and Evans, 2015).

A further ethical issue when using an inclusive research approach is that it can frequently identify unresolved personal issues of both the co-researchers and the people they interview, in terms of living independently and the lack of support from both informal support networks and formal services. These can be serious concerns which need addressing as a priority with policymakers, taking precedence over dissemination of the research output. Some specific examples are a disparity in welfare benefit assessments, lack of support for health and well-being and limited, supported housing options that need social change to benefit the wider group of people with a learning disability who live independently.

Implications of increased self-confidence and awareness of rights

There can be huge contrasts between the private lives of people with a learning disability and their public strong collective voices in the role of self-advocates and researchers Williams (2011). Some of the Building Bridges research group members have grown in confidence and gained new-found freedom of expression. Some have developed from barely speaking in our group to now being able to present in front of hundreds of people with confidence and also ask questions in seminars. However, this new assertiveness can create a backlash when it threatens the status quo at home. When two emboldened female members challenged their male relations by being more assertive, demanding more autonomy at home, including control of their own money, this led to tensions. In one case, a member was temporarily prevented from attending meetings by her family.

Ownership and anonymity

One of the biggest ethical concerns with inclusive research is the issue of anonymity (Tilley and Woodthorpe, 2011). How do we balance protecting people's identities while enabling them to be proud of who they are and their story, which often include aspiring elements of survival and resilience? In the original research project in 2010, university ethical approval was gained which assured anonymity of the participants. Later, the group members' roles developed to co-researchers, and they chose to write their first report, with no names being mentioned. This led to an article for a practitioner journal, where the group members not only wanted their full names included but also their photographs, indicating personal and collective pride and the desire for acknowledgement. After discussion, a compromise was reached where first names only were used.

Realistic expectations for change

In social research there is much talk of 'impact' and expectations that research should be transformational (Danchev and Ross, 2014). However, academic researchers understand that policy and public attitudes can take a long time to change. This can be hard to understand for researchers with a learning disability and often leads to frustration.

Application/relevance to practice

These findings clearly demonstrate some relatively small changes that could be made to enable people with a learning disability to be more involved in their communities. Without significant relationships, people face isolation and loneliness which can lead to depression and self-neglect (McConkey, Dunne and Blitz, 2009; Waldron, 2010). This in turn can add pressure to social care service delivery and budgets. There are also safeguarding implications; people who are isolated have no one to tell if they are undergoing any personal hardship, or problems such as hate crime. Much has been written about people with a learning disability having a history of cumulative, and frequently overlooked, victimisation, including disability hate crime (Equality and Human Rights Commission, 2011; Mencap, 1999; Inclusion North and Coast 2 Coast, 2008; Richardson et al., 2016). However, there is also a growing awareness of the more subtle exploitation of people with a learning disability by people who befriend them and abuse them, which frequently escalates in severity, referred to as 'mate crime' (ARC, 2012). This typically starts with a person initially making friends with a person who they identify as vulnerable, which then goes on to become an abusive relationship. Victims of 'mate crime' tend to be people with a learning disability and other vulnerable people who live independently and outside of the support of services (ARC, 2012; Money Friends and Making Ends Meet Research Group, 2012; Flynn, 2007).

'Choice and control' for people with a learning disability has been recognised as an agenda needing support and has been a priority for commissioners and providers alike since *Valuing People* (Department of Health, 2001). This is supported by the Mental Capacity Act 2005 which requires that people with a learning disability are assumed to have capacity to make decisions regarding their lives. However, when it comes to forming friendships with people in the community there is evidence that for people who live with paid support, staff undertaking their duty of care can be overprotective, for example with risk-averse policies and procedures and the need to undertake risk assessments, which can stifle the development of friendships (Abbott and McConkey, 2006).

Conclusion

The benefits of inclusive research for both co-researchers with a learning disability and for the depth of knowledge and understanding it can deliver by far outweigh the challenges it created. There needs to be consideration of how to enable genuine disability activism, how to use research to inform campaign work, and even be political, while also helping people to understand that change at a policy level can be complex and take time. Awareness of the ethical issues discussed earlier, and how to manage them, is of paramount importance. More people with a learning disability should have the opportunity to do inclusive research, but this will require their co-researchers to assess the potential challenges and issues and implement appropriate plans. University ethics committees should be willing to accept applications where non-academic co-researchers have contributed to the ethics application, enabling them to be part of every stage of the research process. Finally, as Richardson (2012) suggests, we could see people with a learning disability, with support, having a place at the table on ethics committees in the future.

Activity 2

Write a letter of consent for people with a learning disability to take part in a research study in the role of researchers. This will need to be in the format of easy read, using simple words, a clear simple layout and images to support the text.

Further reading

About inclusive research

Nind, M. (2017). The practical wisdom of inclusive research. *Qualitative Research*, 17(3), pp. 278–288.

Walmsley, J., Strnadová, I. and Johnson, K. (2018). The added value of inclusive research. *Journal of Applied Research in Intellectual Disabilities*, 31(5), pp. 751–759.

Link to the full research study

See www.building-bridges-training.org/research-group

References

Abbott, S. and McConkey, R. (2006). The barriers to social inclusion as perceived by people with intellectual disabilities. *Journal of Intellectual Disability*, 10(3), pp. 275–287.

ARC. (2012). *Safety net project.* [online] Available at: www.arcsafety.net/ [Accessed 28 Feb. 2012].

Barnes, C. and Mercer, G., eds. (2004). *Implementing the social model of disability: Theory and research.* Leeds: The Disability Press.

Building Bridges Research Group. (2014). *Small things that make a big difference.* Sandwell Building Bridges Training.

Building Bridges Research Group. (2016). *Living our lives.* Sandwell. [online] Available at: www.building-bridges-training.org

Chadwick, D., Wesson, C. and Fullwood, C. (2013). Internet access by people with intellectual disabilities: Inequalities and opportunities. *Future Internet*, 5, pp. 376–397.

Chappell, A. (2000). Emergence of participatory methodology in learning difficulty research: Understanding the context. *British Journal of Learning Disabilities,* 28(1), pp. 38–43.

Danchev, D. and Ross, A. (2014). *Research ethics for counsellors, nurses and social workers.* London: SAGE.

Department for Communities and Local Government. (2008). *Digital exclusion profiling of vulnerable groups: Adults with learning disabilities; A profile.* London: Department for Communities and Local Government.

Department of Health. (2001). *Valuing people: A new strategy for learning disability for the 21st century.* London: The Stationery Office.

Department of Health. (2010). *Making written information easier to understand for people with learning disabilities.* London: Department of Health.

Equality and Human Rights Commission. (2011). *Hidden in plain sight; Inquiry into disability related harassment.* [online] Available at: www.equalityhumanrights.com/legal-and-policy/inquiries-and-assessments/inquiry-into-disability-related-harassment/hidden-in-plain-sight-the-inquiry-final-report/.

Flynn, M. (2007). *The murder of steven hoskin; Serious case review – Executive summary.* Cornwall Adult Protection Committee.

Herron, D., Priest, H.M. and Read, S. (2015). Working alongside older people with a learning disability: Informing and shaping research design. *British Journal of Learning Disabilities*, 43(4), pp. 261–269.

Inclusion Europe. (n/k). *Information for all: European standards for making information easy to read and understand.* Brussels Inclusion Europe with the support of the European Commission.

Inclusion North and Coast 2 Coast. (2008). *Learning disability hate crime: Good practice guidance for crime and disorder reduction partnerships and learning disability partnerships.* London: Home Office. [online] Available at: http://hdl.handle.net/20.500.12389/21351

Kiernan, C. (1999). Participation in research by people with learning disability: Origins and issues. *British Journal of Learning Disabilities*, 27(2), pp. 43–47.

McConkey, R., Dunne, J. and Blitz, N. (2009). *Shared lives; Building relationships and community with people with intellectual disabilities.* Rotterdam: Sense Publishers.

Mencap (1999). *Living in fear.* London: Mencap.

Money Friends and Making Ends Meet Research Group. (2011). *Money, friends and making ends meet final report.* Sandwell Building Bridges Training.

Money, F. and Making Ends Meet Research Group. (2012). Having friends – They help you when you're stuck. *British Journal of Learning Disabilities Special Issue: The Research and Work of Learning Disabled People with Their Allies and Supporters*, 40(2), pp. 83–164.

Mooney, F., Rafique, N. and Tilly, L. (2019). Getting involved in the community – What stops us? Findings from an inclusive research project. *British Journal of Learning Disabilities*, 47(4), pp. 241–246.

Nind, M. (2014). *What is inclusive research?* London: Bloomsbury.

Nind, M. (2017). The practical wisdom of inclusive research. *Qualitative Research*, 17(3), pp. 278–288.

Northway, R., Howarth, J. and Evans, L. (2015). Participatory research, people with intellectual disabilities and ethical approval: Making reasonable adjustments to enable participation. *Journal of Clinical Nursing*, 24(3–4), pp. 573–581.

Oliver, M. (1992). Changing the social relations of research production? *Disability, Handicap & Society*, 7(2), pp. 101–114.

Richardson, L., Beadle-Brown, J., Bradshaw, J., Guest, C., Malovic, A. and Himmerich, J. (2016). I felt that I deserved it – Experiences and implications of disability hate crime. *Tizard Learning Disability Review*, 21(2), pp. 80–88.

Richardson, M. (2012). Reach for the stars. *Learning Disability Practice*, 15(9), pp. 9–29.

Tilley, L. and Woodthorpe, K. (2011). Is it the end for anonymity as we know it? A critical examination of the ethical principle of anonymity in the context of 21st century demands on the qualitative researcher. *Qualitative Research*, 11(April), pp. 197–212.

Tilly, L. (2013a). An enduring sense of loss. *Community Living*, 26(3), pp. 18–19.

Tilly, L. (2013b). "I ain't been bothered to go': Managing health problems in people with a learning disability who live without support. *Diversity and Equality in Health and Care*, 10(4), pp. 223–230.

Tilly, L. (2014). Making end meet. *Learning Disability Today*, Jan/Feb, pp. 14–15.

Tilly, L. (2016). Issues relating to using a co-productive approach in an accessible technology project. In: *Improving social inclusion using NLP: Tools and resources*. Portorož, Slovenia: LREC Workshop, 23 May 2016.

Tilly, L. (2019a). Afraid to leave the house: Issues leading to social exclusion and loneliness for people with a learning disability. *Tizard Learning Disability Review*, 24(4), pp. 168–175.

Tilly, L. (2019b). Experiences of loneliness: People with a learning disability and barriers to community inclusion. In: B. Fox, ed., *Emotions and loneliness in a networked society*. London: Palgrave Macmillan.

Tilly, L. and Building Bridges Research Group. (2015). Being researchers for the first time: Reflections on the development of an inclusive research group. *British Journal of Learning Disabilities*, 43(2), pp. 121–127.

United Nations. (2007). *United nations conventions on the rights of persons with disabilities*. Geneva: UN.

Waldron, L. (2010). In the community but still alone – The wall between them and us. *Community Living*, 23(3), pp. 16–18.

Walmsley, J. (2001). Normalisation, emancipatory research and inclusive research in learning disability. *Disability & Society*, 16(2), pp. 187–205.

Walmsley, J. and Johnson, K. (2003). *Inclusive research with people with learning disabilities: Past, Present and Futures* London: Jessica Kingsley.

Walmsley, J., Strnadová, I. and Johnson, K. (2018). The added value of inclusive research. *Journal of Applied Research in Intellectual Disabilities*, 31(5), pp. 751–759.

Ward, L. and Flynn, M. (1994). What matters most: Disability, research and empowerment. In: M. Rioux and M. Bach, eds., *Disability is not measles: New research paradigms in disability*. Ontario: Roeher Institute.

Watson, N. (2004). The dialectics of disability: A social model for the 21st century? In: C. Barnes and G. Mercer, eds., *Implementing the social model of disability: Theory and research*. Leeds: The Disability Press.

Williams, V. (2011). *Disability and discourse: Analysing inclusive conversation with people with intellectual disabilities*. Oxford: Wiley-Blackwell.

4 Using online surveys to capture health and social care data

Angela Morgan and Nahid Ahmad

Introduction

In health and social care courses there is an emphasis on contemporary issues, which is often where interest is sparked for students, especially where patient and public involvement is needed (van Schelven et al., 2020). This is a good starting point for generating research ideas. Exploiting the technological advances of the digital age in which we live helps to bring alive the study of contemporary issues. This chapter focuses on the use of online surveys and how these can aid research enquiry in health and social care. An online survey is defined as 'one of the most popular data-collection sources, where a set of survey questions is sent out to a target sample and the members of this sample can respond to the questions over the world wide web'.[1]

Whilst online surveys can no longer be considered new, they – along with other virtual methods – are rising in prominence, particularly in the context of the COVID-19 pandemic, which dominated research decisions at the time of conducting the research reported here and also at the time of writing this book.

There are a multitude of web-based survey platforms and tools available which help in the design of a survey. Table 4.1 lists a few which have been extensively used in health and social care. The functionality and usability of these are comparable. They are generally user-friendly, come with survey templates and guidance and

DOI: 10.4324/9781003157724-4

Table 4.1 Examples of survey tools

Survey tool	*Access*
Survey Monkey	Can sign up for free, with up to 10 questions per survey and 25 responses per survey.
JISC Online Survey (formerly Bristol Online Survey)	The online survey tool is designed for academic research, education and public sector organisations.
Qualtrics	If your education provider is not subscribed to this, there will be a personal cost to you.
Voxco	If your education provider is not subscribed to this, there will be a personal cost to you.

generate a hyperlink which enables the survey to be sent electronically, perhaps by copying and pasting the link into an email. When selecting the tool that is right, the main consideration will be the cost implications.

Advantages of online surveys

- Precise project management by one person – useful in your final year project
- Low cost (if any) compared with other survey modes which rely on paper-based questionnaires
- Adaptability – survey closure date can be manipulated to ensure maximum data capture. Helpful when working to tight deadlines
- Associated material such as the research proposal and conceptual definitions for the study can be linked to the survey
- Design flexibility – quantitative, qualitative or mixed; can design for diversity and different learning styles; routing patterns and logic can be used effortlessly for a smoothly functioning survey that is relevant to sub-samples
- Incorrect contact details for respondents are known immediately if using email distribution

- Ensures data security – surveys can be password protected and web servers encrypted and hidden behind organisational firewalls
- Reliability – test–retest between researchers or by piloting with colleagues can be easily achieved before survey goes live
- Automation in data input and handling – automatic data storage and quick download of data set
- Inclusive and potential wide reach of participants through large geographical spread
- Absence of interviewer – no interviewer bias or desirability bias; no interview appointments required. Helpful when accessing busy health and care professionals
- Convenience – respondents can complete survey in their own time and pace; ability to save responses and return to the survey multiple times, so not having to complete in one sitting
- Tracking and real-time access – swift and accessible analysis as responses come in; instils confidence in the data

Disadvantages of online surveys

- Sample selection bias
- Survey fraud – less accountability; no validity to responses (ticking boxes just to finish quickly)
- Limited sampling – inability to reach challenging populations and respondent availability; lack of access to the internet, for example elderly, people with a learning disability, people with physical impairments, blind or those having no digital skills
- Low respondent engagement – respondents can simply delete the email and survey link; having to send reminders
- Absence of researcher – a trained interviewer would be able to probe and clarify responses
- Almost impossible to achieve 100% response rate – response rates are generally low

- Anonymity disallows data removal if respondent wishes to withdraw later
- Not appropriate method for some samples – where respondents are potentially vulnerable; sensitive topics need to be teased out by a skilled interviewer
- Respondents can respond multiple times to a survey thereby skewing the results – unless of course the survey is set up so that respondents are permitted to reply only once

This chapter draws on a recent research project to show how an online survey was used to research the contemporary issue of parental alienation (Morgan, Ahmad and Webster, 2020), a subject highly relevant to those working with children and families, whether in health, social work or social care. Parental alienation can be seen if a child's resistance or hostility towards one parent is not justified and is the result of psychological manipulation by the other parent. Manipulating behaviours include strategies to control or prevent contact, to denigrate the other parent and/or to align the child with the alienating parent. Role distortion occurs between the alienating parent and child, where an unhealthy alliance positions the child as a partner to the parent. The aim of the research was to understand the views and experiences of parental alienation from the sectors of family law, mediation and psychological therapy. The project was also designed to learn about successful interventions which minimise the effects of parental alienation.

Research question: Is there evidence of therapeutic interventions being used successfully to deal with high conflict cases where one parent is exhibiting alienating behaviour?

Why research parental alienation?

In the modern world family systems are diverse, with the number of single parent and blended families on the increase. A third of families in the UK do not contain a couple in a marriage or civil partnership. About 15% of families are single-parent families, and households containing multiple families have increased the most over the last two decades – by 2019, these had increased by three quarters to 297,000 households (Office for National Statistics, 2019). Change in the family system, for example through separation or divorce, is a feature of these modern family types. If managed well, change can be positive and enrich the lives of those involved, especially children (Luckock et al., 2006).

However, if change is characterised by conflict, this can be both painful and damaging. In the case of parental alienation, the child(ren) and the parent who is alienated bear the brunt of this. The field of parental alienation is still a little-known field and the literature shows key gaps in research and knowledge; however, the effects of parental alienation are well documented. It not only affects the relationship between the child and the alienated parent but can have long-lasting impacts on both. For children who are the victims of this form of emotional abuse, the effects can last into adulthood and include mental illness/depression, low self-esteem, substance misuse, lack of trust, low achievement and a range of issues in their own romantic relationships (Baker, 2005; Baker and Verrocchio, 2013; Carey, 2003; Sher, 2015). For alienated parents, the picture is also grim, with them having higher-than-average levels of depression, symptoms of trauma and risk of suicide (Harman, Kruk and Hines, 2018; Sher, 2015). The need for supportive interventions for families undergoing hostile separation is therefore evident.

Using an online survey to gather data

Before providing a rationale for selecting an online survey for the project, it is important to reflect on why other methods were discounted. One method option which could have provided answers to the key question was semi-structured interviews. The advantages of using this method would have been that a more thorough exploration of our participants' views and experiences would have been achieved. However, a key consideration in real-world research is the cost implication both to the funder and the organisation taking part. There was a finite budget and timeline attached to the research and researchers had to balance the project against other key responsibilities. In this instance, these restrictions meant that the team could not commit the time and other resources which would be required to speak to each participant individually (transcription takes approximately 10 hours for a one-hour interview). A focus group method was also ruled out. Although this would not have been as time-consuming as individual interviews in terms of conducting the fieldwork, the coordination would have taken considerably longer than interviews or survey development. The participant burden would also have been greater, as people would have had to attend either in person or virtually at the same fixed time. This risked low engagement and therefore a low response rate (Monroe and Adams, 2012).

The online survey method was selected as it suited the limited budget and scope of the research and could also be conducted in a short timescale. Other considerations were also better met by using an online survey: the project needed views from participants in multiple locations across the UK, and the research team was also working from three different locations, so the project was being remotely governed by the project manager.

The research process

Online surveys, like any method of social science research, are used to gather data about a topic of interest, analyse these data and synthesise them into results which are presented as research findings in engaging ways. When embarking on a research project where an online survey method is needed, researchers should ensure that the method is suited to answer the research aims and questions. There are five main components to creating an online survey which were all followed during the course of the project:

1. Planning – the topic of interest was researched with the research questions being suitably answered through this method.
2. Designing – the appropriate survey tool was selected (JISC) and questions input, ensuring different response types were considered.

3. Reliability testing and piloting – the survey should be able to measure what it is intended to measure and that it was user-friendly.
4. Distribution – the survey was piloted for functionality and sense-checking, before distributing to the sample.
5. Reporting – analytics and export functions were used to summarise, describe and analyse findings, before presenting them in meaningful ways.

The research plan

The JISC Online Survey tool was selected for the research purpose as the institution has a subscription and so there was no cost to the project. The quality of the results of any survey depends mainly on the implementation of the survey including sensible sampling methods, tool development and proper administration. So, achieving a good quality survey was reliant on understanding the importance of the planning stage. While online surveys allow the creation and editing of a series of questions, it can be difficult to complete this process directly into the software the first time it is used. For this reason, the survey questions were developed in advance, which then made for ease of inputting the questions online.

Design and question response types

Online survey platforms do not have a spellchecker; so, using a Word document, a series of questions was pre-prepared, then edited and arranged in order, making sure there was a logical flow. Next, answer choices were determined for each question.

The survey included a mix of different question types. Closed or forced-entry questions were included so that respondents could only give one answer from a list of pre-set responses, although these single-response questions had different layouts, tabulated and linear. The advantage of this type of question was that the analyst was able to generate statistical data such as whole numbers or percentages and visually represent a summary of all responses. Multiple response questions were also included to allow respondents to choose more than one answer from a list of possible answers. Such questions also included 'none of the above' or 'all of the above'.

Some questions were designed for open-ended or free-text responses. Open-ended questions required narrative responses or in-depth views and experiences (qualitative data) to provide a deeper understanding of responses to closed questions. Respondents were given freedom to share their views in their own words.

Character limits were set for the length of narrative responses in order to control the amount of qualitative data for analysis purposes. This allowed a richer interpretation whilst keeping the data output manageable, where the analyst examined the responses and summarised the key themes. This was more time-consuming than the quantitative analysis, so a careful balance between these two types of questions was applied.

The survey also asked for demographic information at the end of the survey, that is, questions that requested personal information about respondents such as their age group, gender, employment role, etc., as this information could have actually linked well to the research aim. All responses to demographic questions were optional for data protection purposes. Responses to these questions were used for subgroup analysis.

Logic was constructed in the process of creating the survey. Logic, in the context of an online survey, means the ability to skip over certain questions or sections and continue at a future question or section. For example, if a respondent answered a question saying they had experience of someone who deliberately kept their child away from the other parent, then they were directed away from the next few questions which asked more detailed questions about this. An example of survey logic that was applied in the research discussed here later can be found in Appendix I.

There were some questions that the project required respondents must answer, so the survey was designed so that responses to those questions were required in order to progress through the survey. This ensured that data generated was meaningful in answering the research question.

Once the survey had been designed, the questions were reviewed again from the view of those responding to it. For example, did each question flow logically from the previous one and onwards to the next?

Were clear instructions provided? Could those with low literacy skills or who have a learning disability access and complete the survey easily? Was it written in plain English? Could those for whom English is a second language understand it easily? Given the multicultural society we live in it is essential to be aware that key concepts written in English are well understood by speakers and writers of the language in which the survey is designed to be used (Ustün et al., 2003).

Pilot testing

When the team was satisfied with the questions, it was time to test it through a pilot stage. For any survey, designers need to aim to have the best instruments and measures to ensure it is fit for purpose, has good measurement properties and that it has passed through a pilot testing phase to ensure its feasibility. There will usually be a facility within online platforms, such as a flow chart, for previewing the question set and its flow. Pilot testing acts as a 'dummy run' and should take only a few days. Pilot testing the functionality ensured, for example, whether the logic worked and whether the forced responses prevented progression through the survey if unanswered. This meant that where responses to each question were 'required' or 'optional', double checking took place.

Effort was given to examining the data gathered to ensure the survey was fit for purpose or whether changes were needed. Three colleagues were asked to respond to the survey and sent the hyperlink where they could access it. The resultant data were reviewed and 'respondents' were asked for their views on the usefulness of the survey from their perspective. Were there any problems with data entry? Did the questions make sense and apply to their work settings? Were there any gaps in what they would have liked to have seen included? Fortunately, in this instance, there was no need to revise the survey.

Distribution: sampling and recruiting

Once the survey had been piloted, it was ready to go 'live'. There is a facility to include the start and end date on JISC which was used, the survey was made live for four weeks during the summer of 2020. The survey was distributed across England and Wales by email with a participant information sheet to 59 organisations and individuals known for their professional standing in the sectors. The sample was developed from professional networks and organisations and individual practitioners identified through a literature review. However, there were very few responses during this window, so the survey was extended for another two weeks. A total of 29 responses were received.

Reporting and analysing

All online surveys have the ability to see how (anonymised) individual respondents answered all questions as each respondent will automatically be allocated a unique identification number. They can also generate bar and pie charts to provide simple visualisation of data. There is also an inbuilt mechanism to download the data set as a portable document format (pdf) and export the data into a spreadsheet. Data were both quantitative and qualitative and were analysed using descriptive statistics and thematic analysis – no charts were used in the research report as the number of responses was small. For the same reason, the full data set was downloaded as a pdf for ease of analysis.

Reflections on ethics and other considerations

During the planning stage we had to consider the pros and cons of our chosen method, in particular, how well it would allow us to answer the research question in the time frame we were allowing. This had to be revisited once the pandemic reached crisis point in the UK, in terms of how feasible it was to continue as planned. We had to also consider carefully the potential ethical concerns related to the research, especially confidentiality and anonymity.

The research proposal was written prior to the onset of the COVID-19 pandemic. Once the project was underway it became ever more apparent that the pandemic would soon reach the UK, which would create conditions for the volatility of the wider economic, health and social conditions. Given the changes to the UK infrastructure and social movement restrictions during the lockdown which began in March 2020, we had to ensure that it was still feasible to place research demands on the already stretched health and social care workforce. The result of this was the practical issue of trying to secure a good-enough sample size by effective recruitment, whilst ensuring undue burden was not placed on potential respondents (for example by too lengthy a survey, too short a deadline for responses and number of reminders sent).

The low survey response rate is likely to have been due to the impact of the pandemic, with much of our population of interest having moved from centralised offices to working from home, plus organisational preoccupation with supporting the development of online services for practitioners which would have taken priority over requests for research participation. A higher response rate might have been achieved under different circumstances. Certainly, as far as survey distribution was concerned, the sudden move to home working made it difficult (sometimes impossible) to make direct contact with the relevant people in those organisations we were relying on to distribute the survey – we also had the added concern of not wanting to place undue burden by continued 'chasing'. Contact by email provided limited opportunity to ensure that we were reaching the right people at the right time for effective distribution.

Research outcomes: lessons learnt

There were, however, slightly better outcomes as a result of the pandemic. Current restrictions in the context of the COVID-19 pandemic presented perhaps fewer challenges for social care values in that participants were enabled to share their views anonymously in a field that is highly charged with emotion – and during a time when face-to-face methods were not feasible. It enabled individual empowerment and voice in a forum that was confidential and secure. It also allowed for ease of completion through standard tick box questions, whilst also allowing narrative responses in open-ended questions.

The main challenge for this study lay in the inability of many individuals and organisations to respond due to the overwhelming pressures of work that the pandemic had caused, which resulted in a less-than-expected response rate. Another external pressure came through the need to adhere to research governance processes in other

Table 4.2 The link between the research process and findings with health and social care values

Health and social care values	*Research process and findings*
Dignity and respect – spend time listening to people to get to know them and their needs; respect people's right to make their own choices and decisions; communicate with people in a clear, open and straightforward way using appropriate language.	The survey was developed in plain English, avoiding jargon, and most questions were made with an optional response as opposed to a required response. The report was written in plain English, with clearly defined conclusions and recommendations.
Working together – offer people a range of realistic options and choices; be committed to working as part of a team and support others in the team; understand and respect that other people have different priorities and needs.	The corporate response from Cafcass was accepted as it was the only realistic option available to them, and it was incorporated into the findings. The research team comprised multidisciplinary researchers including academics, researchers, a therapist and mediator and every decision taken was done so unanimously.
Commitment to quality care and support – give people your full attention and help people when they need it most; be warm, kind, reliable, empathetic and compassionate towards others; be flexible and react calmly to whatever happens, making changes as necessary.	This was achieved by swift and effective communication between the research team and prospective respondents, answering queries as they arose. Acceptance was shown towards the difficulties experienced as a result of the pandemic and the team remained flexible in the way respondents wished to take part, reminding them that participation was voluntary and there was no compulsion to participate.
Learning and reflection – accept and think about any feedback you are given about your work and learn from the feedback; be honest and transparent and do not be afraid to admit when you have made a mistake; know your own limits and can identify when you need help and support and are feeling stressed by your work.	The research team met frequently to update on progress, risk assess the project, support each other's contribution and consider formative feedback on survey implementation and findings. We asked the funder for comprehensive feedback on a 'headlines summary' of the literature review and the draft report and was prepared to make amendments where required. The whole research team offered and accepted both academic and pastoral support throughout the project, the latter in relation to the pandemic.

organisations. For example, after following this process for the Child and Family Court Advisory and Support Service (Cafcass), we were advised that in the current climate it would not be possible for them to disseminate the survey to its members to complete individually due to their high caseloads. In the event, we received a corporate response which, whilst important in terms of statutory context, was actually meaningless in answering our research question, as what we required for the research was to learn the views and opinions of individuals who follow Cafcass guidelines in dealing with parental alienation.

Nevertheless, insight was gained that added value to what is already known in the field of parental alienation. Table 4.2 shows how the research process and findings link to health and social care values. In a professional context, the survey findings should help to make future health and care decisions, show what has and has not worked well from both a service-user and patient perspective as well as a management perspective and inform future health and social care strategy and service delivery.

Relevance to practice

The research was disseminated in the January 2021 edition of *Parental Alienation International*, the published bimonthly newsletter of the Parental Alienation Study Group (PASG). The report was subsequently disseminated internationally through the PASG wider networks. At the time of writing this chapter, a paper was being written for *Seen and Heard*, the quarterly journal of the National Association of Guardians Ad Litem and Reporting Officers (Nagalro). By seeking to publish in this journal, we hope our research will be read by children's guardians, family court advisers and independent social workers who work with children, parents and carers in family court proceedings.

The low survey response rate was insufficient from which to draw firm conclusions and recommendations, although an attempt to draw insights was made. For instance, the findings showed evidence for the need for reform of the UK family court system, in order to significantly reduce the potential for the courts and legal processes to exacerbate existing conflict and harm to children caused by alienation.

One recommendation included considering amending the widely used Domestic Abuse, Stalking and Honour Based Violence (DASH) risk assessment to identify, where children are affected by domestic abuse, if they are also subject to parental alienation behaviours.

The findings indicated that more research is needed on social workers' and family court advisors' understanding of parental alienation and what interventions they are aware of both outside and inside of the family court system. Knowledge of how they experience and deal with allegations or issues of alienation, the strength of evidence they rely on, their perceived impact of alienating behaviours on children and training needs would help inform education and practice development.

Given the opportunity to run this research differently, future proofing and adaptability to the unpredictability of wider economic, health and social conditions should be considered more thoroughly. Whilst this is always an issue when developing a risk assessment for research, during a pandemic where only virtual methods could be used due to changing social restrictions, it is difficult to think of an alternative virtual method that would have produced a higher response rate. The unprecedented nature of the pandemic also meant that it would have been difficult to predict anything of this magnitude in a risk assessment.

Further, colleges and universities that provide education and training for students preparing to take on roles as health and social care practitioners are an ideal training ground for learning the research process, both in the classroom and in placements. In these courses, the skills learnt will have real relevance for both the future careers of these students and in contributions to wider society. For health and social care students, acquiring research skills is therefore not just about passing courses: it is about making a difference in the real world, which is after all the motivation for those entering these professions. The final year project or dissertation of an undergraduate or apprenticeship course often brings about anxiety and trepidation for students at its mere mention. However, it should be viewed as an opportunity for students to get excited about research. Excitement comes from the selection of a topic meaningful to the student and further enquiry into this topic in order to plan, design and execute a method which generates findings of real interest. Often, this is the beginning of further, more sophisticated research for students, either in postgraduate education and training, or in future job roles. It is the first opportunity a student has to really make their study their own.

Activity 1

Consider this online survey and what you might have done differently, if anything. Think about the different kinds of families as outlined earlier in the section that explores why parental alienation is an important subject for research: couples with disabilities; same-sex couples; ethnic diversity and mixed-race families; one or both parents with a mental health disorder or alcohol/drugs issues, cultures where honour-based violence exists, or domestic abuse. What about other family members such as grandparents?

Activity 2

Imagine you are a children's social care worker. Your manager wants to know the experiences and opinions of social care staff in the region about how they have managed implementing new regulations for children in care: they want the information within the next four weeks. Your colleague suggests you run a survey. So, your task now is to design a set of questions for a survey that you think will give your manager the information they need. Select an online survey tool of your choice and develop your survey by using closed questions, questions with multiple choice responses, questions which require Likert-scale answers and open questions requiring a narrative response. Consider what is reasonable in terms of completion time for busy health and social care staff. Do not enable the survey to go live, but pilot it as discussed earlier. Consider whether to revise your questions.

Note

1 www.questionpro.com/blog/what-are-online-surveys/.

References

Baker, A.J.L. (2005). The long-term effects of parental alienation on adult children. *American Journal of Family Therapy*, 33, pp. 289–302. https://doi.org/10.1080/01926180590962129.

Baker, A.J.L. and Verrocchio, M.C. (2013). Italian college student reported childhood exposure to parental alienation: Correlates with well-being. *Journal of Divorce & Remarriage*, 54, pp. 609–628. https://doi.org/10.1080/10502556.2013.837714.

Carey, K.M. (2003). Exploring long-term outcomes of the parental alienation syndrome. *Dissertation Abstracts International: Section B: The Sciences and Engineering*, 64(5-B), p. 2381.

Harman, J.J., Kruk, E. and Hines, D.A. (2018). Parental alienating behaviors: An unacknowledged form of family violence. *Psychological Bulletin*, 144(12), pp. 1275–1299.

Luckock, B., Lefevre, M., Orr, D., Jones, M., Marchant, R. and Tanner, K. (2006). *Teaching, learning and assessing communication skills with children and young people in social work education*. Bristol: The Policy Press.

Monroe, M.C. and Adams, D.C. (2012). Increasing response rates to web-based surveys. *Journal of Extension*, 50(6), Article number: 6TOT7.

Morgan, A., Ahmad, N. and Webster, M. (2020). *The clinical and legal management of parental alienation in the United Kingdom*. Research report. Wolverhampton: University of Wolverhampton. [online] Available at: http://pasg.info/app/uploads/2021/03/Morgan-et-al.-2020-PA-in-UK.pdf.

Office for National Statistics (ONS). (2020). *Child emotional abuse in England and wales: Year ending March 2019*. London: Office for National Statistics.

Sher, L. (2015). Parental alienation: The impact on men's mental health. *International Journal of Adolescent Medicine and Health*, 29(3), pp. 98–104. https://doi.org/10.1515/ijamh-2015-0083.

Ustün, T.B., Chatterji, S., Mechbal, A. and Murray, C.J.L. (2003). The world health surveys. In: C.J.L. Murray and D.B. Evans, eds., *Health system performance assessment: Debates, methods and empiricism*. Geneva: WHO.

van Schelven, F., Boeije, H., Mariën, V. and Rademakers, J. (2020). Patient and public involvement of young people with a chronic condition in projects in health and social care: A scoping review. *Health Expectations*, 23(4), pp. 789–801. https://doi.org/10.1111/hex.13069.

Link to the full research study

Morgan, A., Ahmad, N. and Webster, M. (2020). *The clinical and legal management of parental alienation in the United Kingdom.* [online] Available at: http://pasg.info/app/uploads/2021/03/Morgan-et-al.-2020-PA-in-UK.pdf.

Further reading

Callegaro, M., Manfreda, K.L. and Vehovar, V. (2014). *Web survey methodology: Research methods for social scientists*. London: Sage.

Woodall, K. and Woodall, N. (2017). *Understanding parental alienation: Learning to cope, helping to heal.* Springfield, IL: Charles C. Thomas.

Appendix I

Survey logic

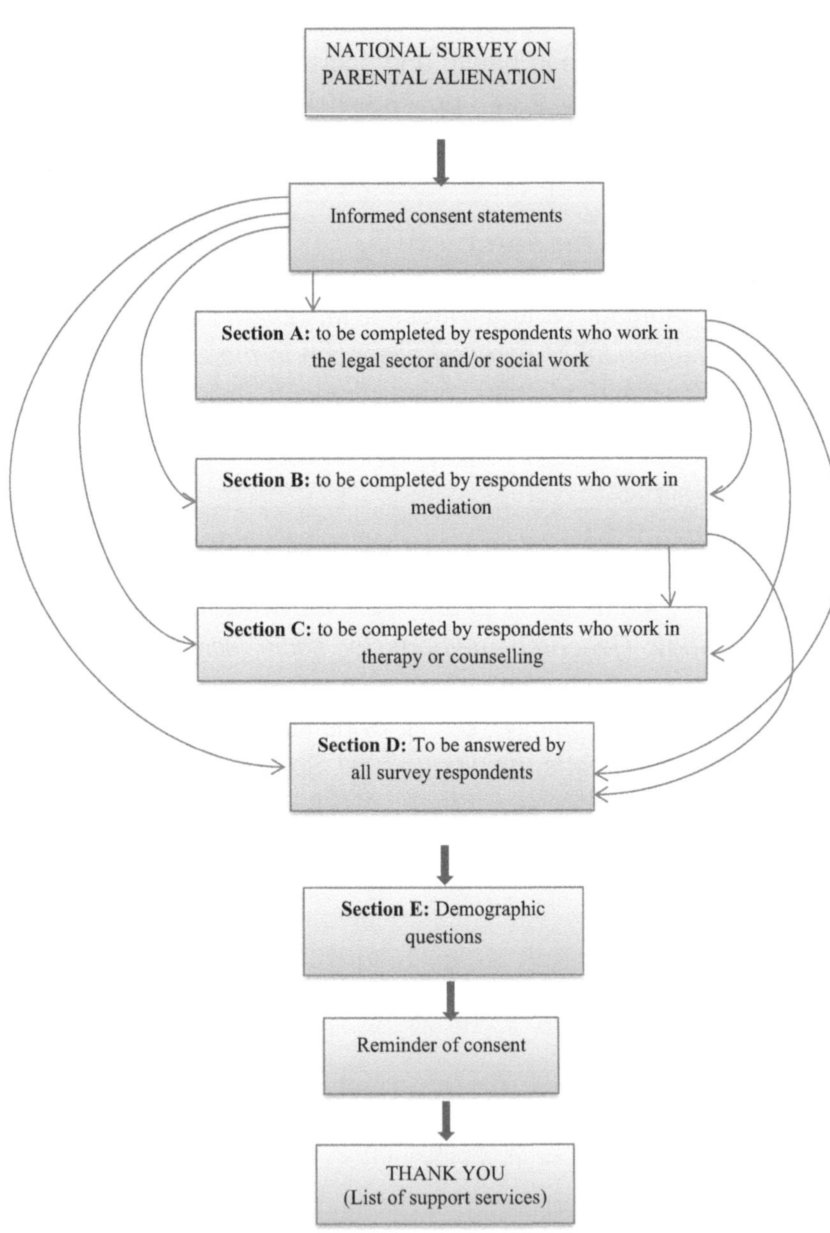

5 Using interviews and focus groups to investigate the effectiveness of mentoring in a UK healthcare trust

Jenni Jones

Introduction

Background to the study

Mentoring in the workplace is becoming more popular than traditional training interventions as it is more personal and tailored to the individual and ultimately is proving to be a cost-effective way of embedding long-term movement and change in an organisation's culture and operations. Essentially, mentoring is a unique interpersonal relationship between two people (Eby, Rhodes and Allen, 2010; Janasz et al., 2013). The key purpose of mentoring relationships is to support and challenge both parties towards their learning and development (Garvey, 2014; Parsloe and Wray, 2016).

Professional nursing has suffered from educational, recruitment and retention challenges over the last decade, and it has since been recognised that role socialisation and career development are a useful ongoing development process (to both the employer and the employee) that can lead to greater job satisfaction and commitment within the workplace. Using a more experienced person as a 'supervisor of practice' to guide and support the less experienced nurses within a 'mentorship' scheme has been the cornerstone of this initiative both in the UK and beyond (Papastravrou et al., 2010.) Mentoring is also being offered in a healthcare setting for other groups;

DOI: 10.4324/9781003157724-5

high potential staff, those new to management and those in transition (NHS Leadership Academy, 2021a).

Based on the understanding that mentoring is increasingly used in a healthcare setting and is seen to benefit both individuals and organisations, this research was aimed at investigating WHAT is being learnt within mentoring relationships within the four established domains of learning (Wanberg, Welsh and Hezlett, 2003; Hezlett, 2005) of cognitive learning, skills-based learning, affective-related (inner) learning and social networks for both parties, WHAT are the moderating factors that help and hinder the mentoring relationship and HOW do both these factors change over time?

Three case study organisations were researched originally but for the purposes of this chapter, the focus will be on the healthcare study. This case study organisation was a UK healthcare trust which involved two large hospitals covering over 500,000 patients and approximately 6,000 employees. To further support their managers, the Learning and Development Department decided to launch a pilot formal mentoring programme to support both clinical and non-clinical members of staff in their part-time study for a postgraduate management qualification.

Research questions

1. What do mentees and mentors perceive they are learning during their formal mentoring relationships?
2. How does the learning change over time for both parties?
3. What are the factors that moderate (help and hinder) the mentoring relationship for both parties?
4. How do these moderating factors change over time?

Research approach and methods used

Semi-structured interviews and focus groups were used for this study.

The aim of this study was to understand the subjective world of the human experience (Cohen, Manion and Morrison, 2017) by uncovering and appreciating the many different realities and meanings that mentees and mentors have created based on their mentoring interactions, whilst taking into account the influence of the organisational context (Bryman and Bell, 2015; Cohen, Manion and Morrison, 2017; Easterby-Smith, Thorpe and Jackson, 2018.)

Recognising that this research was aimed at better understanding the perceptions of people in an attempt to offer 'explanation, clarification and demystification' of formal mentoring, it was decided that a qualitative approach would be best fit for this research. All qualitative and case study methods of data collection were considered for this study including observations, documentation including diaries, archival records, physical artefacts, interviews and focus groups, and it was decided to use both interviews and focus groups; recognising that it was important to hold face-to-face conversations with the people involved to get a deeper sense of their reality.

Interviews

An interview is a 'conversation with a purpose' (Maykut and Morehouse, 2005, p. 75), not unlike mentoring. Yin (2018) suggests that interviews are an essential source of case study evidence and should be 'guided conversations' rather than being too formal and structured. There are a variety of interviews: structured, unstructured and semi-structured (Gillham, 2001). Structured interviews use a predetermined set of questions, they can be administered relatively quickly, and the interviewee's response can be easily coded. Unstructured interviews tend to be more informal whereby the interviewer sets the topic, but the interviewee sets the agenda. For this type of interview, the researcher goes in with a more open mind than structured interviewers might. Semi-structured interviews, used in this study, are a combination of the two aforementioned interviews, whereby the interviewer presents a semi-structured list of themes or questions and has freedom to probe and follow up throughout. There is still a clear sense of the topics to explore and a sense of order in which to explore them, but there is less chance of 'pigeon-holing' the respondents at the outset (as may occur with structured interviews).

According to Gillham (2001), semi-structured interviews are the most important type of interview in case study research. Semi-structured interviews allow consistent themes and questions to be explored (see Table 5.1). Not having a completely fixed framework to follow allows the researcher not to get too 'tied up' (Easterby-Smith, Thorpe and Jackson, 2018) in the formal structure and so allows some flexibility between interviews for further probing and discussion, depending on the attitudes and opinions expressed in the conversational flow (Bryman and Bell, 2015). It was felt that busy people within healthcare may prefer to meet and reflect on events face to face, away from their daily work practices. Meeting people individually gave an opportunity for both the researcher and the mentees/mentors to build a rapport and an element of trust between each other, reiterate and share any questions and concerns about confidentiality, share feedback and be reassured by others. This was also the preference of the sponsoring organisations.

Activity 1

Think of at least one follow-up question for each of the eight aforementioned questions. Remember these are questions used as part of a semi-structured interview process, so there is room to be flexible within them with additional, probing questions to dig deeper.

Table 5.1 Semi-structured interview questions used

Semi-structured interview questions used for both mentees and mentors
• How would you describe your mentoring relationship so far? • What have been your most effective/least effective mentoring experiences? • What do you think you are learning, from being involved in mentoring? • What do you think your mentee/mentor is learning from being involved? • How do you think you and your mentee/mentor is learning this? • What do you and your mentee/mentor do that helps/hinders your learning? • What other factors enable or inhibit your learning whilst mentoring? • What do you feel has changed since you started being involved in mentoring – that is, for you, your mentee/mentor, within the relationship, your job?

Focus groups

Focus groups, like interviews, are about a 'free flowing', but focused, discussion on a particular topic (Fisher, 2010) and have become an important technique because they offer a way for researchers 'to listen to the plural voices of others' (Denzin and Lincoln, 2003, p. 384). It was hoped that those involved in mentoring would be willing to engage in a number of focus group discussions with colleagues, as they may see this as a chance to meet like-minded colleagues and to share similar challenges. It is also a professional requirement for mentors to attend regular 'supervision' type sessions (EMCC Guidelines on Supervision, 2016) to share their ideas, get support and ultimately aid their personal development.

In contrast to interviews, the researcher takes a more marginal role within focus groups, acting as facilitator or discussion stimulator but not as a director or guide. The 'unstructured nature' of the interaction between focus group members helps to take the emphasis off the researcher, as facilitator, and so helps to reduce the influence of their views on the group, thus adding to the objectivity and limiting any bias and subjectivity (Denzin and Lincoln, 2003.) However, it is recognised that the focus group environment is still in some part contrived and involves 'steered conversations' (Easterby-Smith, Thorpe and Jackson, 2018) giving less opportunity for personal responses and issues to be explored in greater depth. There is also concern about the joint production of meaning, as there may be some social or status pressure or dominance from others that may constrain or influence contributions.

Due to the flexible and free-flowing nature of both interviews and focus groups, they were deemed to be the most appropriate data collection methods for this study. The advantage of using two qualitative methods – interviews and focus groups – is that they both provided insights into how the research participants viewed the world. Being present at both, the researcher had some control over the data collection whereby they can follow up areas of interest and probe for further information or clarification to provide more complete, rich data.

Sample and recruitment

The cohort studying the postgraduate qualification were invited to be part of the mentoring programme. As such, this mentoring pilot started with six mentors and six mentees; six dyads but one pair did not carry on their mentoring relationship after a short period of time (and so their results were not included in this study); so only five dyads stayed actively involved in the research throughout. Dyads were made up of three female pairs, one male pair and one female mentee and one male mentor pair.

All mentors and mentees who offered to be involved with mentoring and this research were volunteers. Mentors were all experienced managers, and most were or had been previous students doing the same qualification. Some mentors had mentored or been mentored before. The mentors were trained by an external training company, and once the training was completed, mentors had a group discussion with the Trust Learning and Development team to discuss their expectations, and myself as the researcher, before starting their mentoring relationships. The researcher was not involved in the mentor training nor the mentee matching but was invited to evaluate the programme from the beginning to the end.

In short, ten employees from five pairs volunteered to be part of the study, from either a clinical and/or non-clinical background, across two hospitals. Once the mentoring had started, semi-structured interviews were carried out with each mentor and mentee (except one mentor was working abroad so was not available for the last two interviews) making an overall total of 38 interviews. These 30-minute semi-structured interviews were carried out over a 12-month period at four points to coincide roughly with the four phases of the mentoring lifecycle (Kram, 1988). For instance, interview 1 – at the end of the initiation phase (3-month point); interview 2 – at the end of the cultivation phase (6-month point); interview 3 – at the end of the separation phase (9-month point) and interview 4 – at the end of the redefinition phase (12-month point).

Meeting this homogeneous group at regular intervals allowed the researcher to build a deeper relationship with the mentors and mentees over time and so gain a richer picture of their experiences (Silverman, 2020). The researcher was given the contact details of all mentors and mentees and made her own appointments to meet both parties. There was no Mentoring Co-ordinator involved in setting up the interviews; so, the researcher was in control of coordinating who to meet and when.

Two focus groups were also carried out with mentors only (at the 3-month point and 6-month point) to share challenges and best practice, to discuss the results so far and to gather any additional information. These were organised by the Mentoring Co-ordinator. These were offered as 'supervision' CPD 'giving back' group sessions to support the mentors, so they were not offered to mentees.

Each set of interviews and focus group sessions were recorded and transcribed and then coded through NVIVO software to search for patterns and themes. An overview report was sent back to the management team of the sponsoring organisation. This was also sent to the mentors and mentees to verify the summary and for additional comments.

Activity 2

It is often hard to quantify the impact of activities that involve people developing personal insights, like mentoring, coaching, training, etc. Considering that both mentors and mentees developed an increased confidence over time through their mentoring relationships (linked to the affective-related domain), how do you think you could measure the application of this back in the workplace?

Key findings

Table 5.2 shows a very brief summary of the key findings coming from both the interviews and the focus groups combined.

Table 5.2 Key learnings from the NHS mentoring case study overall, covering all four research questions

Summary of the key findings
• Both parties learn in all four learning domains. • Mentoring develops confidence. • Mentoring develops wider knowledge. • Mentoring develops different skills. • Social networks generally created the least amount of learning. • Affective-related learning increases over time. • Confidence increases over time for both parties. • Cognitive and skill-based learning fluctuates over time. • Additional (facilitating) moderating factors included other (supportive) relationships, similarities and differences. • Managers can be facilitating or hindering in mentoring. • Time is a hindering factor in mentoring. • The pattern of some responses over time was similar for mentees and mentors. • Mentoring seemed to endure and learning occurred despite some significant hindering factors.

These findings, when compared to the other two case study organisations, provided valuable insights towards a better understanding of how to create and nurture formal mentoring as a development tool in the healthcare workplace.

> Mentoring perhaps is an 'unsung hero' in the field of development. Its potential is huge, and with careful planning and a lot of support, can be impressively effective. Innovative mentoring programmes, properly resourced and supported, should be on every HR and Organizational Development team's agenda.
>
> (Western, 2012, p. 53)

Reflections and evaluation of the research study

Hindering factors

The key practical issues and challenges centred on availability, workload, location and bird flu.

All mentors and mentees were initially keen to get involved and were aware of the purpose of the research and their part to play within it. Informed consent was obtained (Bryman and Bell, 2015). However, when it came down to putting a date in the diary for the first face-to-face meeting, this was difficult to do with unpredictable shift patterns and changing rotas. As the research took a longitudinal approach, it was imperative to keep talking to the same pairings at the same intervals throughout the study, so as the researcher I needed to be very flexible with when/where I met the mentees/mentors. I was also conscious of adding to the workload of already busy healthcare practitioners, especially as they were both working and also studying for postgraduate degree alongside. As a result, I chose their coffee/lunch break to meet them and always bought them a coffee as a small token of thanks. It was not an option to arrange video call type meetings as the technology was not available for individual use at the hospitals.

The dual location of the hospitals was also a factor to be navigated when agreeing the days/times to meet, as I needed to schedule this around my own working-day commitments and location of where I was working.

Bird-flu was both a positive and negative factor. On the one hand it meant that those who I was interviewing were now extra busy dealing with the effects of bird flu and so were potentially less available for meeting up. It also meant that they were in the workplace more. This made getting a date in their diary a little easier, albeit needing to meet the participants at sometimes unsociable hours in their longer working days.

The fact that the focus groups were already planned in and considered a mandatory part of the mentoring programme helped to ensure that the mentors protected this time in the diary and were all able to come long.

Facilitating factors

When the mentoring offer was made to the participants, I was there to answer any questions about mentoring but also to explain my role as the researcher. This helped them to see my role was directly connected with the programme and helped me to connect myself with the group very quickly. So, recruiting the sample was easy enough to do, but as it was only a small sample it was crucial to keep the relationship and momentum going with both parties. One pairing did drop off over a short period of time, but once the first interviews were carried out and the first focus group too, a rapport was established with the mentees and mentors which meant that it was easier to keep in touch and build the trust from then on.

Doing a longitudinal study helped to develop a greater sense of what was going on and a better understanding of the organisational culture. In addition, sharing coffees and sitting (most often) in the canteen area created a more relaxed, informal atmosphere in their own surroundings. This not only helped the flow of conversation in the interview but also gave a greater sense of the context and culture of their workplace.

Facilitating the focus groups was also helpful as it created a dynamic within the mentor group that helped to develop a 'community' of mentors who were keen to hear about each other's experiences which again was helpful information for the ongoing research. It also gave me an opportunity to give back to the group by sharing some additional insights to support their mentor training and their CPD.

Ethical issues

There were no ethical issues in relation to this research project.

Sound ethics are the essence and underpinning of good mentoring (Passmore, 2021). Throughout this research, it was extremely important to remain sensitive to the impact of the researcher and this research on those who are approached for help, those who provide access and cooperation and those affected by the results. Maylor and Blackmon (2005) suggest that an overriding ethical principle when researching should be that we treat others as we wish to be treated ourselves and as a result, provide benefits to the individuals and organisations that are involved.

Formal ethical approval was given by the case study organisation through the Mentor Co-ordinator. Once this was attained, ethical approval was sought and given by the university's Research Ethics Committee. Formal ethical approval was not needed through the NHS Trusts (Medical) Ethics Committee as it was clear through the methods chosen that no patients were directly involved, there was no intrusion on their privacy, and they were not affected by the research. Information about participant rights was fully discussed with all mentors and mentees and consent forms were signed by all parties before the research commenced.

All participants were informed through an initial meeting about the aims, purpose and likely publication of findings involved in the research, the potential uses to which the data might be put and any potential risks or consequences for participants. All participants had the right to participate or not, and those that did were clear about the parameters and the purpose. All participants freely gave their informed consent based on a full and fair explanation of the study (Cohen, Manion and Morrison, 2017).

Having face-to-face interviews and focus groups gave the researcher the opportunity to reiterate aspects of informed consent and also to reassure that any personal information concerning research participants was being kept confidentially and anonymised throughout. Any references to names, initials and jobs were removed in the notes that were typed up and shared, to ensure no one could be identified by a third party. Also, permission was sought from all involved to share an anonymised summary of the information with senior organisational stakeholders and later through external publications.

The researcher is a professional member of The European Mentoring and Coaching Council (EMCC) and as such abides by the EMCC Global Code of Ethics (2018) in terms of working with clients, professional conduct and excellent practice. Sensitivity, integrity and confidentiality were maintained throughout.

Reflections on the methods used

Table 5.3 Key advantages and disadvantages of the two methods used

Methods	*Advantages*	*Disadvantages*
Semi-structured interviews	• Can reiterate ethics • Personal account • Rich/deeper information • Could buy a 'thank you' coffee • Flexibility with diary • Freedom to probe beyond set questions • Room to develop rapport and trust	• Time-consuming • Participants' availability • Participants' accessibility • Dual location of hospital • Potential interviewee bias • Potential interviewer bias
Focus groups	• Can reiterate ethics • Quick way of getting a sense of what is going on • Helps to see key themes/patterns • Perceived as a mandatory part of the programme by mentors, so mentors protected time in their diaries to do this	• Still a 'steered conversation' – potential interviewer bias • Can limit personal responses/less detail • Potential 'group think' – go with the majority • Social/status pressure from group • Unable to access mentees too

Application/relevance to practice

The key values of the NHS constitution (2021b) are focused on involving everyone, improving lives and working together. This is essentially and directly the same for mentoring. Table 5.4 shows how the six NHS values can be directly translated into mentoring.

These six values can also be translated into the research process.

1. Working together in partnership; the research was set up with the researcher in partnership with the NHS Trust Learning and Development department, the mentors and the mentees.
2. Respect and dignity; ethical approval was sought and agreed to ensure that everyone who was part of the research was treated rightly and fairly. Mentors were trained so that they could treat their mentees with respect and dignity too.
3. Commitment to quality relationships; the researcher developed quality relationships over time, through the regular interviews.

Table 5.4 The six NHS values and mentoring

NHS constitution (2021b)	*NHS constitution (2021b) translated into mentoring*
1. **Working together for patients**	1. Working together in partnership
2. **Respect and dignity**	2. Respect and dignity
3. **Commitment to quality of care**	3. Commitment to quality relationships
4. **Compassion**	4. Compassion
5. **Improving lives**	5. Improving lives
6. **Everyone counts**	6. Everyone counts

Mentor training and the support given through the focus groups/supervision type sessions helped to secure the quality of the mentoring relationships too.

4. Compassion; this was shown by the researcher in relation to the flexibility and commitment to meeting up regularly. This was also shown by both the mentors and the mentees and evidenced through the feedback shared over time.
5. Improving lives; the results have been shared and this type of mentoring support expanded within and beyond this NHS Trust, which has ultimately touched many lives. The support offered to the mentees was aimed at improving their chances of success with their postgraduate management qualification and ultimately in their management role. The mentor also benefits from this two-way relationship in relation to their learning gained and further skills developed.
6. Everyone counts; everyone who was within this sample group was invited to take part and all their views were equally recorded and taken into account though the interviews and the focus groups.

In addition, mentoring builds in time for reflection on practice for both parties, which in turn enhances knowledge, competence and skills in the role and confidence to make changes. It encourages people to work and learn together and to feel empowered to make changes back in the workplace, which will have a positive impact on all service users. This sits well with the notion of reflective practitioners within the healthcare context too.

In addition, all those involved were either established managers (mentors) or those new to management (mentees), so encouraging managers/leaders to role model (NHS Leadership Model, 2021), share their experience with others and develop mentoring skills as part of their management skills toolkit will have a snowballing effect towards developing more nurturing managers/leaders into the future.

Dissemination

From a research point of view, this research has been disseminated as a report on the NHS Trust involved, through the PhD researchers, through two published articles (Jones, 2012; Jones, 2013) and also contributed to a chapter in a more recent book (Hatton, 2019). More details follow;

Hatton, K. (2019). Developing coaching skills to support OD skills for leaders. In: R.G. Hamlin, A.D. Ellinger, and J. Jones, eds., *Evidence-based initiatives for organizational change and development*, Vol. II. IGI Global, Chapter 21.

Jones, J. (2013). Factors influencing mentees' and mentors' learning throughout formal mentoring relationships. *Human Resource Development International*, 16(4), pp. 390–408 https://doi.org/10.1080/13678868.2013.810478.

Jones, J. (2012). An analysis of learning outcomes within formal mentoring relationships. *The International Journal of Evidence Based Coaching and Mentoring*, 10(1), pp. 57–73. http://ijebcm.brookes.ac.uk/documents/vol10issue1-paper-05.pdf.

Impact on social care/nursing/public health practice, policy or education

From a practical point of view, this research has informed practice about the benefits of mentoring and how best to implement and sustain an effective programme within this NHS Trust and beyond. The learning has been shared and others have come forward to support the initiative. As a result, it has since been adapted into a more formalised coaching programme offered to all employees, rolled out across these two hospitals and also led to a 'coaching skills for leaders' course to enhance all managers' skills set. The impact of these interventions, over a five year period, has since been measured and discussed in a follow-up chapter (Hatton, 2019) which points out that through a survey of the 300+ employees who had been involved, 90% felt it had developed helpful skills for their management and leadership role and 100% of those involved would recommend a mentoring or coaching programme to others. Over 1,000 employees have now accessed some form of coaching or mentoring, representing approximately one fifth of this NHS Trust. As mentioned earlier, more skilled managers and leaders will mean more supported and nurtured teams, which will in turn will mean happier employees and ultimately better supported and nurtured patients.

Further reading

McGrath, C., Palmgren, P.J. and Liljedahl, M. (2019). Twelve tips for conducting qualitative research interviews, *Medical Teacher*, 41(9) pp. 1002–1006. [online] Available at: www.tandfonline.com/doi/full/10.1080/0142159X.2018.1497149.

NHS. (2016). *Running focus groups for patient and public engagement.* [online] Available at: www.england.nhs.uk/wp-content/uploads/2016/07/bitesize-guide-focus-groups.pdf.

NHS. (2020). *Leadership academy on coaching and mentoring in the NHS.* [online] Available at: www.leadershipacademy.nhs.uk/resources/coaching-register/.

Saunders, M., Lewis, P. and Thornhill, A. (2018). *Research methods for business students*, 8th ed. London: Pearson. [Some helpful chapters on doing interviews and focus groups.]

References

Bryman, A. and Bell, E. (2015). *Business research methods*, 4th ed. Oxford: Oxford University Press.

Cohen, L., Manion, L. and Morrison, K. (2017). *Research methods in education*, 8th ed. London: Routledge.

Denzin, N.K. and Lincoln, Y.S., eds. (2003). *Collecting and interpreting qualitative materials*, 2nd ed. London: Sage.

Easterby-Smith, M., Thorpe, R. and Jackson, P.R. (2018). *Management research*, 8th ed. London: Sage.

Eby, L.T., Rhodes, J.E. and Allen, T.D. (2010). Definition and evolution of mentoring. In: T.D Allen and L.T. Eby, eds., *The Blackwell handbook of mentoring: A multiple perspectives approach*. Sussex: Wiley-Blackwell, pp. 7–20.

EMCC. (2016). *Guidelines on supervision*. European Mentoring and Coaching Council website. [online] Available at: www.emccouncil.org/src/ultimo/models/Download/7.pdf.

EMCC. (2018). *Global code of ethics*. European Mentoring and Coaching Council website. [online] Available at: https://emccuk.org/Public/Accreditation/Global_Code_of_Ethics.aspx.

Fisher, C. (2010). *Researching and writing a dissertation for business students,* 3rd ed. Essex: FT Prentice Hall/Pearson Education Ltd.

Garvey, B. (2014). Mentoring in a coaching world. In: E. Cox, T. Bachkirova, and D. Clutterbuck, eds., *The complete handbook of coaching*. London: Sage, pp. 361–374.

Gillham, B. (2001). *Case study research methods*. London: Continuum.

Hatton, K. (2019). Developing coaching skills to support OD skills for leaders. In: R.G. Hamlin, A.D. Ellinger, and J. Jones, eds., *Evidence-based initiatives for organizational change and development*, Vol. II. IGI Global, Chapter 21.

Hezlett, S.A. (2005). Protégés learning in mentoring relationships: A review of the literature and an exploratory case study. *Advances in Developing Human Resources*, 7(4), pp. 505–526.

Janasz de, S., Behson, S.J., Jonsen, K. and Lankau, M.L. (2013). Dual sources of support for dual roles: How mentoring and work-family culture influence work-family conflict and job attitudes. *The International Journal of Human Resource Management*, 24(7), pp. 1435–1453.

Jones, J. (2012). An analysis of learning outcomes within formal mentoring relationships. *The International Journal of Evidence Based Coaching and Mentoring*, 10(1), pp. 57–73. http://ijebcm.brookes.ac.uk/documents/vol10issue1-paper-05.pdf.

Jones, J. (2013). Factors influencing mentees' and mentors' learning throughout formal mentoring relationships. *Human Resource Development International*, 16(4), pp. 390–408. https://doi.org/10.1080/13678868.2013.810478.

Kram, K.E. (1988). *Mentoring at work: Developmental relationships in organizational life*. London: University Press of America.

Maykut, P. and Morehouse, R. (2005). *Beginning qualitative research: A philosophical and practical guide*. London: The Falmer Press.

Maylor, H. and Blackmon, K. (2005). *Researching business and management*. Hampshire: Palgrave Macmillan.

NHS. (2021a). *Leadership model*. [online] Available at: www.leadershipacademy.nhs.uk/wp-content/uploads/2014/10/NHSLeadership-LeadershipModel-colour.pdf.

NHS. (2021b). *Values of the NHS constitution*. [online] Available at: www.healthcareers.nhs.uk/working-health/working-nhs/nhs-constitution.

Papastravrou, E., Lambrinou, E., Tsangari, H., Saarikoski, M. and Leino-Kilpi, H. (2010). Student nurses experience of learning in the clinical environment. *Nurse Education in Practice*, 10(3), pp. 176–182.

Parsloe, E. and Wray, M. (2016). *Coaching and mentoring – Practical methods for improving learning,* 3rd ed. London: Kogan Page.

Passmore, J., ed. (2021). *Excellence in coaching – The industry guide,* 4th ed. London: Kogan Page.

Silverman, D., ed. (2020). *Qualitative research,* 5th ed. London: Sage.

Wanberg, C.R., Welsh, E.T. and Hezlett, S.A. (2003). Mentoring research: A review and dynamic process model. In: J. Martocchio and J. Ferris, eds., *Research in personnel and human resource management*, Vol. 22. Oxford: Elsevier Science, pp. 39–124.

Western, S. (2012). *Coaching and mentoring – A critical text*. London: Sage.

Yin, R.K. (2018). *Case study research and applications: Design and methods*, 6th ed. London: Sage.

6 Making sense of complexity

Using thematic analysis to understand the role of the foster carer

Colin Watt

Introduction

Although the existence of children and young people who display harmful sexual behaviours had been known about in the UK since the early 1990s (Hackett, 2004), surprisingly few studies existed in 2010 (and even today) which described either how those who were unable to live within their own families fared in foster placements or how foster carers responded to the challenges they presented. Such children and young people were (and are) being placed with foster carers and they and their foster carers were (and are) reporting their experiences, in formal review processes, to their supporting social workers and to each other. At the time when this study was planned however, most of these accounts, and the lessons they contained, remained within confidential case files and in looked after children's review reports. This meant that understanding about what happened within placements, and crucially, whether what happened actually reduced the risks these children and young people presented others, or met their own needs, was not shared widely.

DOI: 10.4324/9781003157724-6

This study then was an attempt to answer the following questions:

Research questions

- How do foster carers who look after young people who have sexually abused experience and understand their role?
- How do young people who have sexually abused experience foster care and understand the role of their carers?

The intention in undertaking the research was to find out what both groups thought was good and bad about placements, what was helpful and unhelpful, what 'worked' and didn't work and whether there was any agreement between them about this. It was hoped that findings might lead to the development of a practical 'theoretical framework' with which to better conceptualise foster care for those young people who are known to have sexually harmed others, so that understanding between those providing and receiving services might improve and that what can make a positive difference in these young people's lives might be recognised and shared.

Ethical issues, sampling, recruitment and methodology

As this was always intended to be an initial, exploratory study it was planned that no more than five carers and five young people would be interviewed and that only experienced carers and older young people who had had both successful and less successful placements would be recruited. The reason for this was that it was thought that these would be more likely to have reflected on their own experiences and therefore to be able to offer considered views and opinions.

The particular young people recruited to the study then were those who were in, or had been in, foster care and who had previously been identified, by either criminal justice or public protection processes as having committed sexual offences or as having presented, what was understood to be a definite risk of sexual harm to others. These young people then were either those whose names were on the 'sex offenders' register' or who had been identified as fulfilling 'local multi – agency public protection arrangements' (MAPPA) criteria at level 2 ('those who present significant risk of harm to others'). Foster carers recruited to the study were those who had looked after young people fulfilling these criteria.

The method planned to encourage participants to talk about their experiences was the 'semi-structured interview'. This is a tried and tested way of enabling people to express their 'opinions, feelings, emotions and experiences about sensitive and personal matters' (Denscombe, 2010, p. 174), and it was also the communication style most familiar to the practitioner-researcher from his professional practice. As many people find it difficult or embarrassing to discuss sexual behaviour (and particularly their own harmful sexual behaviour) very careful planning was required and agreement sought with potential interviewees about which subjects would be discussed and which would not.

While it was necessary then to be clear with everyone that the focus of the study was the foster carer's role in caring for young people who had sexually abused (and therefore that each young person taking part had sexually abused), it was not necessary or appropriate, to discuss with young people the sexual behaviour that had brought them into foster care. Young people and carers knew in advance then what they would be asked to discuss and understood that they would not have to discuss anything which made them feel uncomfortable.

Following detailed planning, and ethical approval (from the university supporting and overseeing the study, and from my employing agency), potential participants were identified and recruited. Participants agreed to take part in the project after full and detailed discussions about the purpose and methods of the study and about their rights to anonymity throughout the research process.

In total, six carers and three young people took part in the research, and all described themselves as 'white and British'. None of the young people were connected in any way with any of the carers and all the young people who took part were male and over the age of 18 years (though they described their experiences of being in foster care as younger teenagers).

The interviews were audio recorded so that they could be transcribed and then interpreted or 'analysed'. 'Analysis' here meant taking the 'raw data' from the transcribed interviews and organising them into meaningful groups or categories representing particular concepts that were thought relevant to the enquiry. Data which had something in common, or were similar to each other in some way, were grouped into initial 'codes' and reviewed against descriptive concepts. If these made some sort of sense, and proved consistent through comparison and testing, these codes were then organised into broader units of analysis or 'themes': first 'sub-themes' then broader 'over-arching themes'. At each level of organisation, data were compared with each other and concepts tested to ensure that they both 'cohered together meaningfully within themes and that there were clear and identifiable distinctions between themes' (Braun and Clarke, 2006, p. 91). Finally, themes were defined and named before being reviewed and retested through discussions with more experienced researchers. Explaining the analysis to others, to test whether it made sense to them, helped to assess whether 'findings' were what Lincoln and Guba (1985) and Hammersley (1992) would describe as 'credible', 'dependable, 'confirmable' and 'relevant' (the criteria of good qualitative research).

The analysis was explained, and findings from the data gathered from the interviews presented, by first writing abridged and edited accounts of the experiences and views of each of the research participants. This was intended to honour their accounts, amplify their individual voices and 'foreground' their particular stories. These accounts used direct quotations from the interviews and were presented in sections corresponding to each of the interviews which, when combined, represented views (about foster care with young people who have sexually abused) from 'inside' six foster placements. The first three sections presented the experiences, views and opinions of each of the foster caring couples interviewed and the second three, those of the young people about their own experiences of placements.

The mechanism of analysis of the accounts that provided a view of these foster placements from the 'outside' was then described. This analysis was the researcher's own interpretation of the stories heard and his attempt to identify whether these could be contained within a single conceptual framework that would accurately capture and describe the role of foster carers who look after young people who have sexually abused.

The details of the interpretation and organisation of data, described earlier as 'thematic analysis', is outlined in Table 6.1.

Table 6.1 shows the three levels of interpretation that followed the initial gathering and transcription of data. Extracts from interviews are shown here to demonstrate the initial coding of that data and its organisation within different categories and sub-themes. The underlined extract, from a young person's interview about one of his placements, was interpreted then as evidence both of his understanding of his carers' 'acceptance' of him and of their skill in 'engaging' him within the placement. These terms describe both initial codes and sub-themes (underlined here) which were interpreted as constituting aspects of the *Enabling* key theme.

The italicised extract, from one of the interviews with a foster carer concerning their experiences of looking after a young person, was interpreted as an example of imposing limitations, managing risks, ensuring safety, restricting and supervising. These descriptions were organised within the sub-themes described as providing safety and security and of controlling and interpreted finally as evidence of both *Protecting* and *Constraining.*

The first of three essential elements of the caring role identified by this process of thematic analysis then is that of '*Protecting*'. This theme broadly encompasses both the identification and the management of risks within placements and suggests that, as part of their role, foster carers must anticipate, recognise, understand and attempt to reduce risks of harm to each young person placed with them, as well as to themselves and to others. This, participants described, involves establishing and maintaining appropriate boundaries and providing supervision of the young person whilst in placement. Protecting here is conceptualised as encompassing the

Table 6.1 A summary of the thematic analysis of data obtained from carers and young people describing the role of the foster carer in looking after young people who have sexually abused

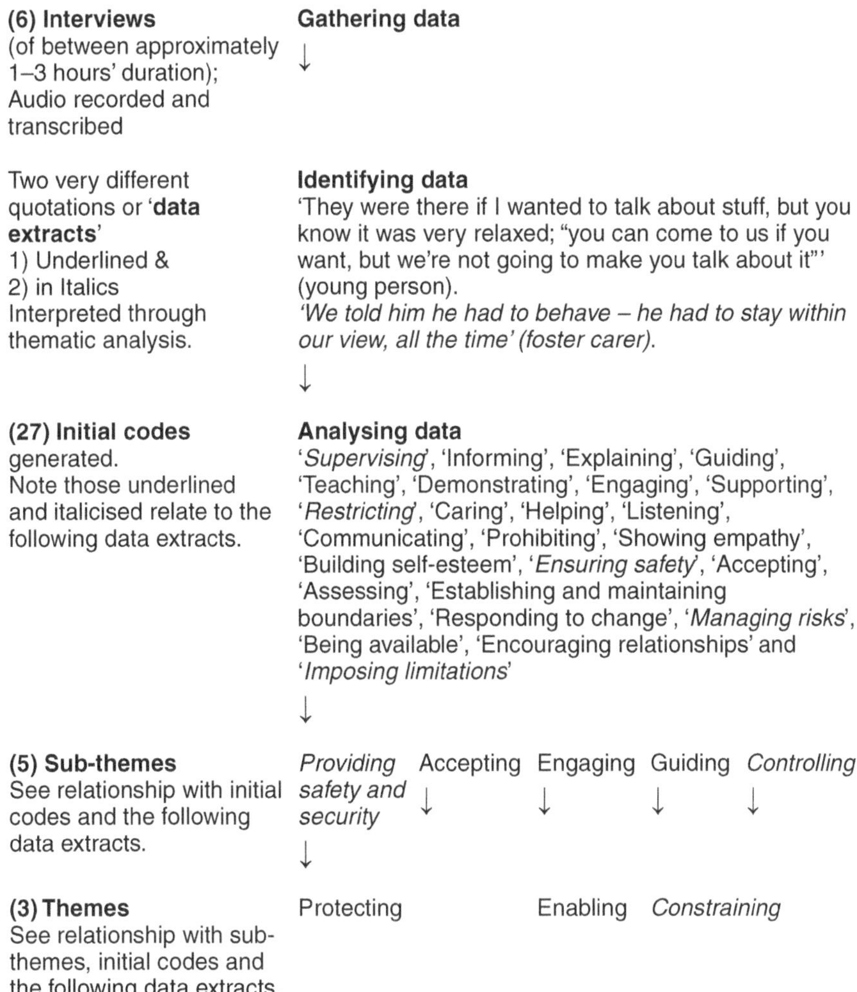

(6) Interviews (of between approximately 1–3 hours' duration); Audio recorded and transcribed	**Gathering data** ↓				
Two very different quotations or '**data extracts**' 1) Underlined & 2) in Italics Interpreted through thematic analysis.	**Identifying data** 'They were there if I wanted to talk about stuff, but you know it was very relaxed; "you can come to us if you want, but we're not going to make you talk about it"' (young person). *'We told him he had to behave – he had to stay within our view, all the time' (foster carer).* ↓				
(27) Initial codes generated. Note those underlined and italicised relate to the following data extracts.	**Analysing data** '*Supervising*', 'Informing', 'Explaining', 'Guiding', 'Teaching', 'Demonstrating', 'Engaging', 'Supporting', '*Restricting*', 'Caring', 'Helping', 'Listening', 'Communicating', 'Prohibiting', 'Showing empathy', 'Building self-esteem', '*Ensuring safety*', 'Accepting', 'Assessing', 'Establishing and maintaining boundaries', 'Responding to change', '*Managing risks*', 'Being available', 'Encouraging relationships' and '*Imposing limitations*' ↓				
(5) Sub-themes See relationship with initial codes and the following data extracts.	*Providing safety and security* ↓	Accepting ↓	Engaging ↓	Guiding ↓	*Controlling* ↓
(3) Themes See relationship with sub-themes, initial codes and the following data extracts.	Protecting		Enabling	*Constraining*	

physical and emotional safety of the young person cared for and of others, and as aiming to increase everyone's actual, and felt, safety and security.

The second essential element of the caring role identified through this analysis is defined as '*Enabling*'. This encompasses a broad range of sub-themes describing parenting and pedagogical tasks, including the provision of physical and emotional care, information giving, explaining, guiding, teaching and demonstrating. It also includes categories identifying less defined activities such as engaging, accepting and supporting. Collectively, these seemed to be understood, by carers and young people, as helping the young person to acquire and develop skills, overcome trauma and disadvantage and achieve a positive self-identity. Enabling then, is understood by research participants, as promoting young people's health and well-being, equipping them for adulthood and helping them to lead enjoyable and fulfilling lives.

The third main theme identified as an aspect of the role undertaken by foster carers here, is defined here as '*Constraining*'. This describes those interactions between carers and young people which either attempt to control, or are experienced as controlling, through containment and imposition. It suggests actions intended to restrain and inhibit; to restrict choices, limit exploration and curb freedoms. It implies attempts to determine rather than facilitate, steer rather than guide and force rather than encourage.

The relationship between these three core elements is interesting. *Protecting* seemed to be understood by participants either in relation to *Enabling* or to *Constraining*. The young people interviewed then appeared to regard *Protecting* and *Enabling* in very close relationship and almost as interchangeable or synonymous. *Protecting was* enabling for them and *Enabling was* protecting. In contrast while they offered few examples of being constrained by carers, those they did appeared to them, almost the opposite of enabling. They understood that *Constraining* may have been an understandable approach for carers to adopt in response to their past offences, and it may have protected others from them, though in their opinions, it did not provide them, with what they needed in order to grow and develop.

The carers interviewed appeared to perceive aspects of their roles as more distinct. One couple's understanding of the caring role seemed closest to that of the young peoples in that *Protecting* and *Enabling*, if not synonymous, overlapped considerably. They likened looking after a young person placed with them then, to 'holding a child's hand while he learns to walk and picking him up when he falls'. Another couple, in describing how they looked after one particular young person, appeared to regard *Protecting* as more closely related to *Constraining*. They insisted that the only way to ensure the safety of others and to reduce this child's vulnerability was by 'locking him away' or 'supervising him 24/7'. The third couple interviewed seemed to view all three aspects as being in a more dynamic relationship which each other. *Protecting* overlapped more or less with *Enabling* and with *Constraining* depending on circumstances. These carers wanted very much to enable a young person placed with them and to be supported to do this, though they recognised that there were times when they felt it necessary to constrain him and they described being very uncomfortable with this. Eventually, they found the strain in managing the tensions between these aspects of their perceived role, too great and sadly, they resigned from foster caring.

Review and evaluation of the study

So, did the analysis make sense and are these findings 'credible', 'dependable, 'confirmable' and 'relevant'? Has it made some sort of sense of complexity?

I believe this exploratory study achieved a number of aims. It has certainly provided useful data about foster care of young people who have sexually abused. It confirmed the importance of providing opportunities for young people and carers to share their experiences of placements and it demonstrated the significant contribution that service users and practitioners can make to the development of 'knowledge and scholarship' (Shaw, 2005) as well as to the evaluation, planning and development of services (Hackett, Masson and Phillips, 2006). The study showed me that it is possible to gather sensitive data about a challenging and under-researched area of practice in a way which can benefit those who take part, and I believe it has enabled the development of a useful model with which to conceptualise the role of the foster carer in caring for young people who have sexually abused.

Readers though will have recognised some limitations of the study. Principal among these is the very small number of interviews from which data has been gathered. Had I interviewed other carers and young people they would have undoubtedly described different experiences of placements and provided further data with which to explore the questions being asked here and this would likely have allowed me to develop a more comprehensive analysis and perhaps a better understanding of what goes on in foster placements. It would have been helpful then to have interviewed more carers and young people and particularly more carers who had had successful placements and more young people who had experienced unsuccessful placements.

It would also have been helpful to have had an opportunity to test the organisation and interpretation of data offered here through follow-up interviews with the research participants themselves. This might have achieved what Denscombe (2010, p. 299) describes as 'respondent validation' of the analysis and promoted a more participative experience of the research process for those taking part. It might also have provided opportunities to further explore and test the data gathered from initial interviews and to uncover any 'missing' data, perhaps concerning the nature of the relationships between carers and young people. The study undertaken however was the study that was possible for me at the time and with the resources available and while findings from it should be considered in relation to the acknowledged limitations, I believe they raise some important issues for foster carers and for professionals who arrange and support these placements.

First, while it is clear that caring for young people who have sexually abused presents foster carers with particular and significant challenges, I believe this study has shown that these challenges are not insurmountable. Foster care can and does provide some young people who have sexually abused with rich and positive experiences and with the stability and security they need to overcome significant disadvantages and trauma and to enter adulthood successfully (DfES, 2006, p. 3). These findings then provide support for the argument that foster care should remain an option for those young people who have sexually abused and who are unable to live within their own families.

Second, I believe the study has shown that foster carers understand the tasks they undertake in placements very differently. While all the carers interviewed understood that their role involved *protecting* themselves, the young person placed with them and others, they differed in how they thought they could achieve this. Some appeared to think that *protecting* meant *enabling* the young person to achieve developmental goals and independence; others appeared to understand it as involving controlling and curtailing the young person's behaviour in such a way as to *constrain* their development and independence.

The young people who participated in the study also appeared to understand the foster carers' role in these terms. They were clear however that although they had experienced some aspects of their placements as *constraining*, the proper role of foster carers was to *protect them* and others from harm while *enabling* them to achieve developmental goals. This suggests to me a very helpful way of understanding the foster carer's role which if adopted by fostering services might encourage more open and meaningful dialogue with carers and young people about their placements. Effective care of young people who have sexually abused both *protects* and *enables* young people to achieve developmental tasks while less effective care fails to protect and actually *constrains* young people's journeys towards successful independence.

Third, this study has shown me that foster care can only be a viable option for young people who have sexually abused when foster carers are themselves *enabled* and *protected* to *enable* and *protect* young people. Those who support foster carers then need to understand their role in ensuring that placements *protect* and *enable* both carers *and* young people. I think this offers a very helpful way of understanding the role of the supporting social worker which, if adopted, might facilitate a more open and meaningful dialogue between carers and social workers about their foster placements. *Protecting* foster carers involves identifying and minimising risks to them and ensuring they feel safe: *enabling* foster carers involves ensuring they understand both their responsibilities to the young people they look after, and how to fulfil these, while supporting them in their role.

The conceptual framework developed here then describes both the role of the foster carer in looking after the young person and those of the service provider and others in supporting the carer and the placement. This means that it fulfils the last of the tests of good qualitative research suggested by Lincoln and Guba (1985) and Hammersley (1992), that of 'transferability'; the findings can be applied to other contexts and settings.

The 'Protecting, Enabling, Constraining' framework developed (or the PEC model as I have begun to call it) is certainly broad enough to encompass the particular challenges associated with placements involving young people who have sexually abused and to be relevant to foster placements involving young people who have not sexually abused and its use therefore is consistent with the approach that considers these particular young people 'young people who have sexually abused' rather than 'sexual abusers' (Lovell, 2002). It is also, I believe, broad enough to be able to encompass and therefore complement other more established theoretical models describing foster care and the development of sexually harmful behaviour in young people.

Before being adopted more widely further work would of course be needed to explore whether the model can be applied to different types of foster placements ('short term', 'long term', 'emergency', 'respite', 'remand', 'treatment' for example) to placements involving carers or young people from different cultures (and perhaps to placements involving girls and young women who have sexually abused) as well as to understand whether carers and those who support them recognise and understand the developmental tasks young people need to achieve and the specific challenges they face in attempting to do so.

It would be particularly important then to explore further whether carers accept a role in *enabling* the companionable non-abusive sexual behaviour of young people who have sexually abused in the same way as they might accept a role in, for example *enabling* a young person with a physical disability to acquire mobility skills. Carers in this study seemed to understand that they had a proper role in *enabling* young people not to sexually abuse and to support them to manage their sexual behaviour within certain boundaries though they were less clear how they might facilitate young people's positive sexual expression.

Application/relevance to practice

Coulshed and Orme suggest that 'to be truly effective, social workers need to be constantly asking "why?" and that it is in this quest for understanding, that theory informs practice' (2006, p. 9). This project was born out of a desire to better understand the association between theory and practice in social work and to be able to 'defend what we, as social work practitioners, think and do, while remaining open to new ideas and fresh research' (Howe, 2009, p. 205). It provided an opportunity to begin to develop theory and to test this against theoretical models informing practice in foster care and in work with young people who have sexually abused at that time, and it has been a vehicle then to explore the relationship between inductive critical reflection and deductive evidence-based practice. It has shown me that 'practice (including what service users have to say about practice) is a rich source of social work theory and knowledge that complements and enhances formal theories' (D'Cruz, Gillingham and Melendez, 2007, p. 74).

The method used to gather data here proved appropriate to the practice context and to the type of data sought and also to be effective. This represents a significant achievement and offers future researchers a possible template for engaging service users who are often excluded from participatory activities as well as for facilitating discussions about highly sensitive subjects. The main tool used to collect data here was the semi-structured interview with questions providing both triggers and signposts for discussions about specific issues and prompts for clarification. These interviews provided evidence then of participants' prior learning about their experiences of foster care and also of 'learning through reflection' during the interview. Several participants reported valuing the opportunity provided by discussion to explore past events and suggested that these had helped them to make sense of some very difficult experiences.

Research method: semi-structured interviews

These are conversations 'initiated by the interviewer for the specific purpose of obtaining research-relevant information and focussed on content specified by research objectives' (Cohen and Mannion, 1989, p. 307). They require careful preparation and a great deal of skill to work for both parties.

Advantages

They are flexible and adaptable.
They can provide rich data.

Disadvantages

They are time-consuming.

They lack standardisation which means that researcher biases are difficult to rule out (Robson, 2002).

The six foster carers who participated in the study described very different experiences of caring for young people, though they confirmed the nature of the challenges they faced as being to do with understanding and managing the risks of sexual harm they believed those they looked after presented. They understood these risks differently and they approached the management of these risks according to how they perceived individual young people, how they understood their role and how well supported they were by others. Placements were most successful when young people, their carers and carers' social workers shared an understanding about their purpose and when carers were well supported. Placements were most vulnerable, and stalled or broke down, when carers perceived their role differently from those who were supporting them or when the support they received was inadequate. This suggests that foster carers must receive adequate training and appropriate, ongoing support to look after young people who have sexually abused (Sinclair, 2005).

It is important to restate here that this study was conducted ten years ago and that since then, understanding about foster care has developed, professional practice has continued to evolve and legislation has been updated. Following the publication by the government in 2007 of 'Care Matters: Time for Change' and its promise to 'improve the plight of children in care', National Minimum Standards and Regulations for the provision of fostering services were updated (DfE 2011), and in 2017, the Social Work and Children Act required local authorities and their partners to have regard to the 'Corporate parenting principles' (first outlined in 'Care Matters') in carrying out any of their functions in relation to the children and young people they look after. These have been welcome and transformative developments which have both articulated and clarified the roles and responsibilities of all those providing fostering services to children.

Together, they provide a comprehensive and detailed description of the expectations government and society has of its 'corporate parents' and also of how outcomes for children in care are to be improved. My own study represents an attempt to track developing understanding amongst those delivering and receiving foster care at that time of change and to distil the lessons of experiences from within foster placements. I believe the strength of the conceptual framework developed lays in its simplicity and its ability to link the tasks carers perform with actual outcomes for young people. Very simply put, what carers do in *protecting* and *enabling* is to *protect* and *enable* young people; in *constraining*, carers *constrain* young people.

In summary, the strength of this study was that it demonstrated that carers and care-experienced young people have important views and opinions to share about their experiences of placements. Professionals have a responsibility to listen to these, to continue to learn from them and to share those lessons as widely as possible.

Link to the full research study

Watt, C.F. (2014). *"I couldn't understand why anyone would let someone like me into their house": Foster care for young people who have sexually abused.* University of Birmingham. [online] Available at: https://etheses.bham.ac.uk/id/eprint/4778/

Activity 1

Making sense of complexity: analysing a conversation with a friend

- Choose two or three partners (fellow students) with whom to have a 20-minute audio recorded conversation about something you all find interesting (for example 'memories of school', 'first day at college/university' or 'what you would do if you won the lottery').

- Separately, listen to the recording you have made and, using pencil and paper, write notes organising your conversation into categories representing particular aspects of the topic you have discussed.
- As you organise the content of your conversation, identify and name the sub-themes discussed and provide an example of each.
- Identify and name two or three overarching themes in the content of your conversation.
- Discuss and compare your analyses with each other and justify the themes you have chosen.
- Did you all make the same sense of your discussion?
- Compare the analysis of your conversation with that offered by Braun, V., & Wilkinson, S. (2003) discussed in Braun, V. and Clarke, V. (2006) listed in Further reading.

Further reading

About the methodology: Part 3 of Bryman, A. (2016). *Social research methods.* Oxford, UK: Oxford University Press (particularly Chapters 17, 18 and 20).

About the research topic: Hackett, S. (2014). *Children and young people with harmful sexual behaviours.* London: Research in Practice Research in Practice Research Reviews, p. 15.

References

Braun, V. and Clarke, V. (2006). Using thematic analysis in psychology. *Qualitative Research in Psychology*, 3, pp. 77–101.

Braun, V. and Wilkinson, S. (2003). Liability or asset? Women talk about the vagina. *Psychology of Women Section Review*, 5(2), pp. 28–42.

Cohen, L.H. and Mannion, L. (1989). *Research methods in education*, 3rd ed. London: Routledge in Robson, C. (2002). *Real world research*. London: Wiley.

Coulshed, V. and Orme, J. (2006). *Social work practice*, 4th ed. Basingstoke: Palgrave Macmillan in Howe, D. (2009). *A brief introduction to social work theory*. Basingstoke: Palgrave Macmillan.

D'Cruz, H., Gillingham, P. and Melendez, S. (2007). Reflexivity, its meanings and relevance for social work: A critical review of the literature. *British Journal of Social Work*, 37, pp. 73–90 in Howe, D. (2009). *A brief introduction to social work theory*. Basingstoke: Palgrave Macmillan.

Denscombe, M. (2010). The good research guide for small-scale social research projects, 4th ed. Berkshire, England: Open University Press.

DfE (Department for Education). (2011). Fostering Services: National Minimum Standards. Available at: https://assets.publishing.service.gov.uk/government/uploads/system/uploads/attachment_data/file/192705/NMS_Fostering_Services.pdf.

DfES (Department for Education and Skills). (2006). *Care matters: Transforming the lives of children and young people in care*. [online] Available at: https://assets.publishing.service.gov.uk/government/uploads/system/uploads/attachment_data/file/332642/Care_Matters_Transforming_the_Lives_of_Children_and_Young_People_in_Care.pdf.

DfES (Department for Education and Skills). (2007). *Care matters: Time for change*. [online] Available at: https://assets.publishing.service.gov.uk/government/uploads/system/uploads/attachment_data/file/326311/Care_Matters_-_Time_for_Change.pdf.

Hackett, S. (2004). What works for children and young people with harmful sexual behaviours. Essex: Barnardo's.

Hackett, S., Masson, H. and Phillips, J. (2006). Exploring consensus in practice with youth who are sexually abusive: Findings from a delphi study of practitioners views in the United Kingdom and the republic of Ireland. *Child Maltreatment*, 11(2), pp. 146–156.

Hammersley, M (1992). Some reflections on ethnography and validity. *International Journal of Qualitative Studies in Education*, 5(3), pp. 195–203.

Howe, D. (2009). *A brief introduction to social work theory.* Basingstoke: Palgrave Macmillan.

Lincoln, Y.S. and Guba, E.G. (1985). *Naturalistic inquiry.* Beverly Hills, CA: Sage.

Lovell, E. (2002*). 'I think I might need some more help with this problem': Responding to children and young people who display sexually harmful behaviour.* London: NSPCC.

Robson, C. (2002). *Real world research: A resource for social scientists and practitioner-researchers.* Wiley.

Shaw, I. (2005). Practitioner research: Evidence or critique? *British Journal of Social Work*, 35(8), pp. 1231–1248.

Sinclair, I. (2005). *Fostering now: Messages from research, department for education and skills.* London: Jessica Kingsley Publishers.

7 Participatory approaches to building knowledge

Katy Goldstraw and Andrew Beeput

Introduction

This chapter explores the advantages and challenges of using a multi-layered qualitative methodology when researching a health and social care setting. The chapter reflects on the practicalities and ethical challenges of participatory working. It is co-written with the organisation in which the research took place, the Bond Board, and drawn from the findings shared in a previously published project report (Goldstraw, 2018). It seeks to draw out best-practice principles for co-produced creative approaches to participatory research.

Research methodology

A participatory co-produced methodology was key as in addition to the research findings benefitting their organisational strategy the organisation wanted the research process to be emancipatory and empowering for participants (Facer and Pahl, 2017). Using participatory co-produced approaches to researching client needs, the Bond Board was able to develop its strategic direction to align more clearly with client assets. The Bond Board are a not-for-profit organisation based in Rochdale and Oldham, working to reduce homelessness by finding homes in the private rented sector for people on low incomes. The Bond Board worked with individuals and families, offering housing and welfare support and advice to people who were classified as being on level four of the CHAOS Scale (University of the West of England (UWE), 2017). This group of people often have

DOI: 10.4324/9781003157724-7

multiple complex needs and can feel excluded from mainstream services (UWE, 2017). The CHAOS Scale helps to assess people with multiple needs who, despite being ineligible for a range of services, require targeted support. The scale includes engagement with services, self-harm and risk to self and others. Each item in the assessment is rated on a 5-point scale with 0 being a low score and 4 being the highest score. Low scores denote lower needs. The CHAOS assessment is completed by support workers. The research approach was tailored to people who attended a support and advice café and a drop-in centre run by the Bond Board.

The participatory research approach was co-designed with Bond Board tenants, volunteers and employees in order that the research met participant needs. Creative and participatory mapping, interactive activities, participatory workshops and micro semi-structured interviews led by peer researchers formed the data collection methods.

Research question: To understand how to design Bond Board services appropriately in order to promote meaningful engagement

Research methodology

Participatory research

'A research methodology and approach to scientific inquiry characterized by shared leadership among researchers, community stakeholders, and the beneficiaries of research' (Parra-Cardona, Beverly and López-Zerón, 2020).

The HARP project

The main objective of the research was to help the Bond Board to understand how to design services in order to promote meaningful engagement. The research worked with tenants, staff and volunteers to develop the research objectives and to co-design the methodology. Bond Board tenants are described within Bond Board communications as clients and or as service users.[1] How to describe people who access a service is contested. The term client, service user or the term person with care and support needs are often used but have been critiqued as disempowering (McLaughlin, 2009). Sometimes, a Bond Board client might also be a tenant, other times a client might access HARP project services but not be a tenant with the Bond Board. This chapter refers to people who access the Bond Board services as clients.

The Homeless Advice and Resilience Project (HARP), a Big Lottery-funded partnership project delivered by the Bond Board and local partners, invited the Institute for Public Policy and Professional Practice (I4P) at Edge Hill University to work with them. The HARP project worked with excluded and marginalised individuals to provide intensive one-to-one support, short-term crisis solutions, a specialist welfare rights service and offer opportunities for clients to become involved in peer research. A detailed report that summarised the learning was produced, and this chapter draws on text from the report and links learning identified in that report (Goldstraw, 2018).[2]

Understanding the ideas behind the research. Defining participatory co-produced research

Co-produced participatory research challenges power relations, seeking to link research with empowerment, education and action. Participatory research involves research participants in the research process, co-producing knowledge that recognises all people's (community member, citizens, residents, professionals, etc.) power and voice in the community (Evans and Fisher, 1999). Often, 'professionals' or 'academics' hold the voice and power when talking about research. The aim of participatory co-produced approaches to research is that the power is shared, that all members of the research team – client, staff, volunteer and academic – share power and voice and are encouraged to participate on an equal footing. The aim of participatory research in the context of the HARP project was to recognise and empower HARP clients as critical thinkers, who could then engage with the HARP project strategy as empowered individuals.

Activity 1

Pros and Cons Thinking about the participatory co-produced ideals of this research project, what research approaches might you use?

List the pros and cons of these different approaches to the research: focus groups, surveys, interviews and participatory workshops.

Sample and recruitment

A multi-layered approach was used within the research project. This approach combined participatory activities with HARP clients, participatory workshops with volunteers and staff, the training of peer researchers, micro interviews and creative arts activities. Clients were invited to participate in the workshops, participatory activities and semi-structured interviews when they attended the advice café and through staff contact sessions. Staff and volunteers were invited to participate in the research through staff newsletters and internal staff and volunteer communication. Research participation was voluntary, and there were no inclusion or exclusion criteria to allow maximum inclusivity.

Two participatory workshops were held with staff and volunteers. Four participatory activities were held at various times within the project setting to increase participation. Fifteen peer-to-peer semi-structured micro-interviews were conducted. The collaborative analysis was made up of two informal analysis sessions, one workshop with staff and four sessions led by artists at the project setting.

Ethical issues

It is important to consider the ethics of participatory working. The Bond Board client group experience multiple disadvantages. If a person has become homeless or is worried about becoming homeless it can be extremely upsetting and stressful. Often, clients who attend the Bond Board advice café to access housing advice, feel vulnerable, scared and alone. The Bond Board advice café was open to Bond Board existing clients and members of the local community who might wish to become Bond Board clients in the future or simply wish to attend the advice café to socialise. As researchers we hold a duty of care for the emotional and physical health of those involved in participatory and co-produced research (Warr et al., 2016). It was imperative that the research took an ethical approach to working with Bond Board client groups, empowering and supporting HARP clients to develop their voice (Kagan et al., 2017).

Taking an ethical approach to research involves the safeguarding of voice (Wiles et al., 2012), and as such the research data was collected anonymously and informed consent was obtained from HARP clients and the Bond Board. The project itself required and achieved ethical approval from Edge Hill University Ethics Committee. The Bond Board as an organisation signed a detailed research consent form that was displayed in the project setting. Support workers within the setting explained what anonymous involvement in the research involved and supported HARP clients to offer informed consent to anonymous participation. This ensured that the research consent process was explored fully, both verbally and in writing; this was especially important as many clients had limited literacy skills.

The first challenge of the research was to design and deliver participatory activities that could help clients of the HARP project identify and map their strengths. This strengths-based approach is discussed within this chapter as assets. A range of participatory activities that could be used as part of the project sessions were developed. These included participatory mapping of social assets (Putnam, 1995) and of human, financial, physical and public assets (May et al., 2009). To complement and layer the learning from these participatory activities, fifteen peer-to-peer semi-structured micro interviews were conducted. Peer researchers were trained and supported to conduct short five-to-seven-minute interviews with other clients at the centre. These micro interviews worked well. The conversations were undertaken, in the advice café, by joining the table of those to be interviewed and sitting with them while they drank their tea, conversing in an informal manner and asking them about their thoughts in response to the two research questions. HARP drop-in clients responded well to this approach, happy to share their thoughts and experiences.

Micro-interviews conducted in tandem with the university researcher were not in the original plan but they are evidence of the importance of reflexivity in co-produced research and of the need for research flexibility (Dean, 2017). The peer researchers were committed and very keen to be involved. However, using the Dictaphone, attending informal training sessions and building up the confidence to have conversations, as well as remembering the research questions, were a lot to ask of HARP peer researchers. The questions had to be memorised by some researchers as literacy was a challenge for them. After discussion with the peer researchers, it was decided that the university researcher would sit with them as they conducted the interviews, to support them in using the Dictaphone and to help them remember the questions. Taking a reflexive (Dean, 2017) and iterative (Williams and Pierce, 2016) approach to the research was important. Co-produced research needs to share the decision-making power (Facer and Pahl, 2017) and in working collaboratively with communities should respond and adapt to the communities' preferred approach (Kagan et al., 2017).

Two research questions were asked: how do you feel about the advice café? and what top tips would you share with people new to the Bond Board?. These simple accessible semi-structured interview questions opened a conversation with clients and offered an opportunity for clients to respond freely. A range of responses were shared that revealed the range of social, human, financial and public assets that clients could access at the Bond Board.

> I think it's [the HARP project] a good thing it offers support for the tenants cause the majority of the tenants on the bond board you could meet . . . you can socialise you can ask the staff any questions and they will get you an answer. They have council people come down to help with your council tax, rates anything like that.
>
> (Quoted in Goldstraw, 2018)

> Its nice cause we met new people. Yes we usually have a food bag or a cleaning bag. . . . [the HARP project staff] told me about it like and as soon as I got one of their [Bond Board] properties she asked if I wanted to come along like you see then I though id come down. I don't really get out much and I lost my dad in November do I had nothing to you know . . . so I was just stuck in me property but I met [couple sat with] at church. I do go to church and they said come down like. I started coming out now to the coffee morning and it gets me out of the house. Its socialising really and its being able to chat with other people . . . if you've got problems you can ask for help.
>
> (Quoted in Goldstraw, 2018)

> I think it's [the HARP project] a good thing it offers support for the tenants cause the majority of the tenants on the bond board you could meet . . . you can socialise you can ask the staff any questions and they will get you an answer. They have council people come down to help with your council tax, rates anything like that . . . And basically you get a red cross parcel every time so yeah I think it's a good thing really. . . . It gets people out socially.
>
> (Quoted in Goldstraw, 2018)

The research analysis was open and iterative (Williams and Pierce, 2016) in its approach. Key terms and significant issues for the data analysis were identified through a collective contribution process (Datta et al., 2015) by returning to the HARP drop-in sessions for discussion with clients. As this was a piece of participatory co-produced research, it was important that the analysis was co-produced with HARP clients and that they retained control over the data analysis (Datta et al., 2015). The aim of these collaborative analysis sessions was to allow the conversation around client assets to mature and to gather a more nuanced picture of how clients negotiate their assets, and in turn to consider how this could influence and develop the organisational strategy for the Bond Board.

Artists worked with HARP clients, throughout the research process. Artists produced visual images that summarised clients' reflections on their research. These artists were paid professionals and produced a range of visual art from graphic representations of the participatory activities to visual mapping of key themes within the research analysis. These images were then displayed, offering HARP clients the opportunity to have a visual research product; this was especially important for those clients who were unable to read and write (Goldstraw et al., 2020). Working with artists and using creative approaches to co-production was arguably an important approach that held the potential to destabilise traditional power relationships between the university, HARP staff, volunteers and clients (Fullan, 1999). However, it should be noted that artistic approaches alone will not facilitate equality (Foster, 2016), and co-produced participatory approaches must also work hard to build relationships of trust and collaboration (Goldstraw and Diamond, 2018).

Activity 2

Mind Map Using the project summary that you have just read think about what key issues might need to be thought about when designing a project with people who might feel vulnerable and marginalised. Draft a mind map that considers these issues.

Reflection: what worked about the approach taken by the project

Participatory co-produced approaches seek to collaborate, share power and involve genuine participation within the research. The co-produced participatory approaches enacted within the HARP project produced evidence of the power of the voice of people with lived experience within a place (Kagan et al., 2017). There are challenges to this approach: creating safe spaces to share knowledge and addressing power hierarchies within organisational structures are challenging, but the value of enacting social justice by involving those with lived experience of the effect of local, regional and national politics is irrefutable (Vaughan, 2014). In recognising the variety of types of knowledge held by a community there is significant power in co-produced research and how it is represented (Tuhiwai-Smith, 1999).

The research reinforced the importance of developing a safe space for participatory research to happen (Stoudt, 2007). Participatory researchers struggle to build relationships and at times have been critiqued for tokenistic use of client involvement (Sandhu, 2017). It is important to note that this participatory research took place within an already existing project, where clients felt safe and where trusted staff and volunteers worked side by side with clients to support their full participation. Client voice and participation of HARP clients were at the forefront of the research design, activity and analysis. It was essential that the research approach was reflective (Dean, 2017) and iterative (Williams and Pierce, 2016); some approaches worked and others had to be redesigned. The willingness of the HARP clients and the staff and volunteers to be reflective and flexible was fundamental to the co-produced and participatory approach of the project.

The research took a respectful approach to those with lived experience, being clear where their voice could hold impact and where system constraints could present insurmountable barriers to change (Vaughan, 2014). Honesty is important and communities respect that (Cahn, 2000). Developing a safe space for all holds multiple and complex challenges but can also hold opportunities to facilitate clients' voice, enabling them to share lived experience which can in turn influence policy and practice (Stoudt, 2007).

Research relationships were key to the project's success. Building good quality working relationships takes time. By spending time in unstructured interaction, developing working relationships, drinking coffee together and in informal conversation, as well as in more formal training opportunities, working relationships were built that enabled good quality reflection and communication once the peer research began (Head, 2007). The research process involved and included the voices of clients, staff and volunteers. Staff worked with and supported clients to participate in activities and in doing so built on existing strong working relationships. The research took time to involve and listen to staff and volunteers, who then introduced the participatory activities and the university researcher to the space. Staff and volunteers in this sense acted as gatekeepers to the process, signalling that the research was trustworthy, and that the university researcher was a safe person to share stories with. This process was time-intensive yet necessary as working relationships, trust and knowledge take time to build, especially with client groups who have not always had positive dealings with unknown professionals such as university researchers (McDavitt et al., 2016).

Taking an iterative approach to learning

It was important to take a reflective (Dean, 2017) and iterative (Williams and Pierce, 2016) approach to the research, learning from each research interaction where approaches needed to be adapted. Semi-structured interviews usually ask a series of questions and tend to last 30–45 minutes (Guba and Lincoln, 1994). Once the peer-to-peer interview conversations began with the HARP clients, it became clear that long and in-depth discussions were not the best research method to use with a chaotic client group. Addiction and mental health challenges for many clients meant that sitting in one place and concentrating for longer periods were simply too much (Owen, 2001). People attended the drop-in to socialise, to have a cup of tea and some toast and to access advice and welfare support. Clients simply did not want to take part in long conversations. It was therefore decided, on reflection (Dean, 2017), that micro interviews were the best, least disruptive and most accessible approach. These micro interviews worked well. They were five-to-seven-minute conversations undertaken by joining the table of those to be interviewed and sitting with them while they drank their tea, conversing in an informal manner and asking clients for their thoughts in response to the two research questions. HARP drop-in clients responded well to this approach, happy to share their thoughts and experiences.

Activity 3

Top Tips Thinking through the earlier discussion of what worked and what the co-produced approach learnt along the way, develop five Top Tips for co-produced participatory research.

The ethics of practice. Drawing learning, developing recommendations

By reflecting on the co-produced participatory approaches used to empower client voice in this health and social care setting, best practice principles can be developed. These can feed into policy and practice development around client engagement in social care service provision. It is important when taking a reflective approach to learning to be transparent about what worked and where areas of learning have emerged. The research deliberately took a reflective (Lewin, 1951) approach, seeking to reflect the Bond Board's commitment as a learning organisation (Sen, 1991). Recognising research participants as reflexive beings and involving participants in reflexive dialogue during data analysis or evaluation (Dean, 2017) are key to participatory approaches.

The value for health and social care settings of using reflective participatory approaches to research sits in the democratisation of knowledge and the opportunity to build client voice (Curato, Hammond and Min, 2019). Using participatory approaches offers an opportunity for reflection and learning. Alongside this, a strong working relationship between the volunteers, staff and university researcher enabled the research to be flexible and responsive to organisational needs and pressures. The trust and respect held by the staff and volunteers facilitated the involvement of HARP clients in the research and enabled the creation of a safe space (Stoudt, 2007) for involvement.

Time frames were flexible, which facilitated a flexible approach to the project. It is important to remember that truly engaged work with communities takes time, and in taking time it builds the opportunity for informal knowledge and working relationships to be developed (Kagan et al., 2017). On occasions specific safeguarding crises meant that the research had to take a background role in order for clients' immediate needs to (quite rightly) be the focus. The value of time, trust, flexibility and strong working relationships was key to the participatory research work in this health and social care setting.

Key learning messages

Reflecting on the experience of existing participatory and co-produced methodologies within the HARP project, reflective cues for future projects were created as part of the project's learning and are identified on page 44 within the original project report:

Power Co-produced and participatory approaches have a responsibility to negotiate conflicted conversations and to recognise and empower all voices within these conversations.

Ethics Taking an ethical approach to research involves the safeguarding of voice. As researchers we hold a duty of care for the emotional and physical health of those involved in participatory and co-produced research.

Legitimising knowledge Universities hold status and power within the community. Developing participatory and co-produced research validates the universities' commitment to the community and adds an academic status to community-led research. This status can be useful to legitimise community voices and knowledge and to gain funding opportunities.

Conflict Communities are not places of consensus. Participatory and co-produced methodologies need to represent the contested nature of the conversations they hold.

Respect This needs to be established. It takes **Time** and requires **Trust**.

Language Participatory and co-produced research needs to be accessible. The language used within the research process and within any research outputs, for example reports, needs to be appropriate. (Goldstraw, 2018, p. 44)

Conclusion

This chapter has considered participatory approaches to building knowledge, focusing on a case study example of participatory research with a non-governmental organisation, the Bond Board, that specialises in supporting housing needs. A participatory co-produced methodology was key, as in addition to the research findings benefitting its organisational strategy, the organisation wanted the research process to be emancipatory and empowering for participants (Facer and Pahl, 2017). This chapter has described the research methodology and reflected on its success in terms of building client voice and referred to the challenges of co-producing knowledge with people who are living chaotic lives in extraordinarily difficult circumstances (Wall, 2017).

Advantages of research method

- It is strengths based, so builds client empowerment and voice.
- It is flexible and reflective, so can adapt to changing situations.
- It is inclusive of a variety of research approaches from workshops to interviews to artistic involvement.

Disadvantages of research method

- It takes a significant time commitment by researcher and research participants to engage in project and build good quality working relationships.
- It involves complex project management of multiple interlinked research activities.

This chapter has explored the advantages and challenges of adopting a multi-layered qualitative methodology, including reflecting on the practicalities and ethical challenges of participatory working. The chapter is co-written with the organisation in which the research took place, the Bond Board, and has drawn best-practice principles for co-produced creative approaches to participatory research.

Further reading

Participatory & co-produced research methods

Stoecker, R (2013). *Research methods for community change.* London: Sage.

Research report

Goldstraw, K. (2018). *The bond board assets based research project: Final report.* Edge Hill: Institute for Public Policy and Professional Practice.

WEBLINK: www.edgehill.ac.uk/i4p/files/2019/02/FINAL-REPORT-SLA-Bond-BOARD-2018.pdf

Homelessness

Cloke, P., May, J. and Johnsen, S. (2011). *Swept up lives? Re-envisioning the homeless city.* John Wiley & Sons.

Notes

1 www.thebondboard.org.uk/projects/service-user-engagement/
2 Goldstraw, K. (2018). *The bond board assets based research project: Final report.* Edge Hill: Institute for Public Policy and Professional Practice.

References

Cahn, E.S. (2000). *No more throw-away people: The co-production imperative.* Washington, DC: Essential Books.

Curato, N., Hammond, M. and Min, J.B. (2019). *Power in deliberative democracy.* Cham: Palgrave Macmillan.

Datta, R., Khyang, N.U., Khyang, H.K.P., Kheyang, H.A.P., Khyang, M.C. and Chapola, J. (2015). Participatory action research and researcher's responsibilities: An experience with an Indigenous community. *International Journal of Social Research Methodology*, 6(18), pp. 581–599.

Dean, J. (2017). *Doing reflexivity: An introduction.* Bristol: Policy Press.

Evans, C. and Fisher, M. (1999). Collaborative evaluation with service users. In: L. Shaw and J. Lishman, eds., *Evaluation and social work practice.* London: Sage, pp. 11–117.

Facer, K. and Pahl, K., eds. (2017). *Valuing interdisciplinary collaborative research: Beyond impact.* Bristol: Policy Press.

Foster, V. (2016). *Collaborative arts-based research for social justice*. Routledge.

Fullan, M. (1999). *Change forces: The sequel*. London: Falmer Press.

Goldstraw, K. (2018). *The bond board assets based research project: Final report*. Edge Hill: Institute for Public Policy and Professional Practice.

Goldstraw, K. and Diamond, J. (2018). A good society: A critical reflection. *Local Economy*, 33(6), pp. 565–568.

Goldstraw, K., McMillan, A., Mort, H., Pahl, K., Pool, S., Rafiq, Z. and Rasool, Z. (2020). Co-producing artistic approaches to social cohesion. *Research for All*.

Guba, E.G. and Lincoln, Y.S. (1994). Competing paradigms in qualitative research. *Handbook of Qualitative Research*, 2(163–194), p. 105.

Head, B.W. (2007). Community engagement: Participation on whose terms? *Australian Journal of Political Science*, 42(3), pp. 441–454.

Kagan, C., Lawthom, R., Clennon, O., Fisher, J., Diamond, J. and Goldstraw, K. (2017). Sustainable communities: University-community partnership research on social dimensions of sustainable development. In: W. Leal Filho, ed., *Sustainable development research at universities in the United Kingdom*. Cham: Springer, pp. 245–262.

Lewin, K. (1951). *Field theory in social science; Selected theoretical papers*. Edited by D. Cartwright. New York: Harper & Row.

May, C., Brown, G., Cooper, N. and Brill, L. (2009). *The sustainable livelihoods handbook: An asset based approach to poverty*. Oxfam, Church Action on Poverty.

McDavitt, B., Bogart, L.M., Mutchler, M.G., Wagner, G.J., Green Jr, H.D., Lawrence, S.J., Mutepfa, K.D. and Nogg, K.A. (2016). Peer reviewed: Dissemination as dialogue: Building trust and sharing research findings through community engagement. *Preventing Chronic Disease*, 13.

McLaughlin, H. (2009). What's in a name:'Client', 'patient', 'customer', 'consumer', 'expert by experience', 'service user' – what's next? *The British Journal of Social Work*, 39(6), pp. 1101–1117.

Owen, S. (2001). The practical, methodological and ethical dilemmas of conducting focus groups with vulnerable clients. *Journal of Advanced Nursing*, 36(5), pp. 652–658.

Parra-Cardona, R., Beverly, H.K. and López-Zerón, G. (2020). Community-based participatory research (CBPR) for underserved populations. *The Handbook of Systemic Family Therapy*, 1, pp. 491–511.

Putnam, D. (1995). Bowling alone: America's declining social capital. *Journal of Democracy*, 6(1), pp. 65–78.

Sandhu, B. (2017). *The value of lived experience in social change.* [online] Available at: thelivedexperience.org [Accessed 28 Nov. 2018].

Sen, A. (1991). *What did you learn in the world today?* Harvard Institute of Economic Research Working Papers 1536. Harvard: Institute of Economic Research.

Stoudt, B.G. (2007). The co-construction of knowledge in 'safe spaces': Reflecting on politics and power in participatory action research. *Children, Youth and Environments*, 17(2).

Tuhiwai-Smith, L. (1999). *Decolonising methodologies: Research and indigenous peoples.* London: Zed Books.

University of West of England (UWE, Bristol). (2017). *Building connections; Golden key local evaluation. Phase 2. Report* Bristol Leadership and Change Centre, Bristol Business School, April 2017.

Vaughan, C. (2014). Participatory research with youth: Idealising safe social spaces or building transformative links in difficult environments? *Journal of Health Psychology*, 19(1), pp 184–192.

Wall, J. (2017). *Substance misuse and homelessness in greater Manchester.* Lifeline Data Analysis Project, 27 February 2017.

Warr, D., Waycott, J., Guillemin, M. and Cox, S. (2016). Ethical issues in visual research and the value of stories from the field. In: *Ethics and visual research methods.* New York: Palgrave Macmillan, pp. 1–16.

Wiles, R., Coffey, A., Robinson, J. and Heath, S. (2012). Anonymisation and visual images: Issues of respect, 'voice' and protection. *International Journal of Social Research Methodology*, 15(1), pp. 41–53.

Williams, O.R. and Pierce, J. (2016). Iterative parallelism as research praxis: Embracing the discursive incommensurability of scholarship and everyday politics. *Area*, 48, pp. 222–228. doi:10.1111/area.12258.

8 Dialogical narrative analysis of practice-based educators' stories of student placements

Ani Murr

Introduction

Skills developed by designing and carrying out research are valuable not only for becoming a researcher but also for becoming a social care or healthcare practitioner. This is particularly apparent in narrative research, which requires an ability to listen sensitively and attentively to people's experiences. This chapter gives an account of narrative research that explored the stories told by social work practice educators about their experiences of student placements. In social work education, practice educators are social workers who support the learning and assessment of students in practice. This introduction explains how this research into their experiences got its focus and why the approach taken and methods used were suited to its aim.

The original intention had been to focus the research on an examination of practice educators' assessment of social work students' practice during their placements. However, during the pilot study, it was difficult to keep practice educators on the subject of assessment because there were so many other things they wanted to talk about. This brought the realisation that there was a richer vein of their experiences to be explored beyond assessing students. This realisation was strengthened by an argument found in the literature that practice educators' role in helping students learn was not being given

DOI: 10.4324/9781003157724-8

enough attention in education research because of an overemphasis on researching assessment (Domakin, 2014; Woods, 2015). In light of this, the research focus was widened to become an exploration of practice educators' experiences of being practice educators, with the practice educators themselves choosing which of their experiences to talk about. This change of direction in the research illustrates that social research is not a linear process, but it takes twists and turns. This is not unusual and need not be feared.

> **Finalised research question:** What do practice educators' stories reveal about their perception of practice education and their positioning within it?

With its focus widened, the aim of the research became an exploration of what practice educators' stories revealed about their perception of practice education and their positioning within it. The word positioning was used, rather than position, because it could portray the dynamic nature of taking up a position, shifting position or being manoeuvred into a position. As a study that had become more exploratory than explanatory, it lent itself to an interpretivist research design. Interpretivism is concerned with understanding how people make sense of experience: for example, what meanings they ascribe to events and relationships. Interpretivist research recognises that multiple, rather than single, meanings are made from subjective human experience (Creswell, 2018). Narrative enquiry was chosen as the specific research strategy because storytelling is argued to be a significant way in which humans make sense of experience and convey the meaning of their experience to others (Squire, 2008; Bolton and Delderfield, 2018). Narrative enquiry is undertaken in the belief that telling a story about an experience reveals the sense being made of that experience (Riessman, 2004; Hancock, 2016). For these reasons, studying the stories practice educators told was considered a good way of gaining insight into their perception of and positioning within practice education.

So far, the way in which the research got its aim has been explained, along with explanations of why an interpretivist research design was suited to exploring experience and why narrative enquiry was an appropriate strategy for gaining insight into the sense being made of experience. There are many forms of narrative enquiry (Riessman, 2004) and dialogical narrative analysis was chosen for this study (Frank, 2010, 2012). This approach views narratives as broad patterns or templates that stories follow. For example, a pattern for an apocalypse narrative is that there is something which threatens the earth (meteorite strike, volcano eruption); there are people scattered in different places needing to work together to save the earth; efforts to save the earth are jeopardized (sabotage, mechanical failure, unexpected turn of events); people make sacrifices to save the earth; the earth is saved. This overarching narrative can be used to tell many different stories. There are many narratives that shape our storytelling, including quest narratives, rags-to-riches narratives and coming-of-age narratives. While narratives generally shape the way we tell stories, over time the way stories are told can reshape the narrative and new narratives are created. More explanation is given about dialogical narrative analysis after a brief explanation of how the stories to be analysed were gathered.

Semi-structured, narrative interviews were used to gather stories (Cohen, Manion and Morrison, 2011; Jovchelovitch and Bauer, 2000). The interviews were semi-structured in that a loose sequence of questions and prompts was followed. They were narrative in that the questions and prompts invited participants to talk about their experiences; favourite experiences, worst experiences, most difficult experiences and experiences from which they had learnt something. Prompts used in narrative interviewing are designed to encourage storytelling. Examples include, 'What happened next?'; 'Tell me more about'; 'Has something similar happened before?'; 'Can you give me an example?'. Asking 'Why?' is avoided because it can be perceived as threatening or may encourage a participant to give an explanation rather than tell a story (Savin-Baden and van Niekerk, 2007). Once the stories were gathered, dialogical narrative analysis (Frank, 2010, 2012) was used to analyse and interpret them.

Dialogical narrative analysis

Frank (2010, p. 152) defines dialogical narrative analysis as a method of questioning that requires a researcher to think about one story with another story, referred to as thinking *with* stories. It looks for patterns, themes, symmetries and dissonances between stories as if the stories themselves were in dialogue with each other. The purpose of dialogical narrative analysis is to generate a new narrative from the stories; a new narrative that offers fresh understanding of storytellers' problems that helps solve, manage or cope with those problems (Frank, 2010). What this means is explored further in the following.

Dialogical narrative analysis does not follow a step-by-step prescriptive procedure but offers a way of questioning stories that guides analysis and interpretation. Questions central to dialogical narrative analysis include: what do the stories tell us about who the storytellers are? How do storytellers hold their own in their stories? What is at stake in their stories? Derived from these, the following questions were used to address the overarching research question in this study.

- What do practice educators' stories tell us about who practice educators are?
- How do practice educators hold their own in their stories and against whom are they holding their own? (To 'hold their own' means to sustain their worth, as individuals or a collective, against any threats to it.)
- What is at stake in the stories? (This refers to that which is at risk, or in jeopardy, in the stories.)

Responses to these questions were generated by considering (1) how each story depicted the characters in the story, for example angry, frustrated, lazy or passionate characters, 'goodies and baddies'; (2) how trouble was dealt with by a story and how a story might create trouble, for example how problems were explained or explained away, who was blamed for problems and who was exonerated; (3) the extent to which the story presented different points of view and the extent to which it opened up or closed down alternative perspectives, for example whether the storyteller only told their side of a story or whether they mentioned that which other characters might have been thinking or feeling, and whether influences beyond the immediate experience were mentioned; (4) how the story revealed moral complexity, for example how the stories portrayed good and bad practice, good and difficult students, good and poor educators and (5) how each story related to the other stories, for example where they shared common themes, what the different ideas presented were, what contradictory views were apparent. These questions were not mechanistically posed nor did they need to be asked in any particular order. They provided guidance for an attentive and close reading of the stories to aid analysis and interpretation (Frank, 2010, 2012). To support this, I designed an 'initial analysis' template to record key thoughts, an example of which is given in Figure 8.1.

Initial story analysis: participant *X* story *Y*	
Depiction of characters	*Hard working practice educator; poor student; negligent tutor*
Dealing with or creating trouble	*Mistrust of tutor by practice educator, heightened by poor responses from tutor to requests for help. Different priorities for practice placement agency and university.*
Point/s of view offered	*Practice educator's perspective only.*
Interpretive openness	*Although from practice educator's perspective, the practice educator did consider impact on student as well as self.*
Inherent morality	*Good/Bad student support. Giving too much and giving too little support to the student are bad; but the story is trying to make sense of how much is too much? How little is too little?*
Resonance with other stories	*Five other practice educators told stories about the dangers of giving too much and giving too little support to students.*

Figure 8.1 Initial story analysis sheet for dialogical narrative analysis

Sample and recruitment

In this section of the chapter, the participants and how they were recruited is described and an overview of key findings and points learnt is given.

All participants were experienced practice educators working with students studying at the university within which this research was being conducted. Practice educators employed by the university were excluded to avoid a conflict of interests. Purposeful sampling (Cohen, Manion and Morrison, 2011) was used to select experienced, currently active practice educators working in different practice settings across different geographical locations. Invitations to participate were emailed to 12 such practice educators. Each potential participant was sent information about the research that included instruction on what to do if they were willing to be interviewed. Of the 12, five did not reply, one declined and six expressed willingness to participate. It had been thought that ten practice educators would need to be interviewed to generate a sufficient sample of stories, but over 40 stories were gathered from these six practice educators, and this influenced a decision not to recruit further participants.

As explained earlier, the purpose of dialogical narrative analysis is to generate a fresh narrative of participants' experiences that can help them deal with the difficulties they experience (Frank, 2010). Many of the practice educators' stories were about disagreements. Initial analysis of the stories clustered them according to:

1. What the disagreements were about, for example allocation of work appropriate for learning, assessment, suitability of the placement.
2. Who the disagreements were with, for example managers, supervisors, students' tutors.
3. How the disagreements were resolved, for example calmly and collaboratively or angrily and unilaterally.

Key findings from the interpretation of the stories using the method of questioning advocated by dialogical narrative analysis is set out in Figure 8.2.

What do the stories tell us about who practice educators are?	They are boundary workers, working in a complex landscape criss-crossed with boundaries between practice and education.
How do practice educators hold their own in their stories and against whom do they hold their own? Who or what is threatening their worth?	They hold their own using boundary working skills against managers and supervisors in placement agencies and against managers and tutors in universities. These managers, supervisors and tutors frequently undermine their authority, question their jurisdiction and overrule their judgements and decisions.
What is at stake, or in jeopardy, in practice educators' stories?	The recognition, respect and authority of practice educators to fulfil their role.

Figure 8.2 Key findings from the dialogical narrative analysis of stories told

The fresh narrative generated from this interpretation was that practice educators work in a complex landscape of overlapping boundaries that generates disputes about who has authority to make decisions in student placements. Such disputes were identified as jurisdiction boundary disputes. Key learning arising from this was that boundary working skills (Williams, 2011; Oliver, 2013) can be used by practice educators to manage and resolve jurisdiction boundary disputes calmly, collaboratively and cooperatively. I address the implications of this learning for social care and healthcare practice later in the chapter.

Ethical issues

In this section of the chapter, the ethical concerns of the research are considered.

In common with many projects, the ethical concerns of this research were that it should protect the confidentiality of participants and be trustworthy, credible, dependable and confirmable (Cohen, Manion and Morrison, 2011, p. 182). Although the identity of participants can be protected by storing data securely, using pseudonyms and omitting from reports any personal details that could identify them, there remains the possibility in narrative research that individuals are identifiable from the stories they tell. This risk was explained in the information sent to participants and a reminder given in a pre-interview briefing.

Trustworthiness of research needs to be protected when researchers are practitioners in the field of study and known to participants, as I was in this research. The trustworthiness of the research was protected by being transparent and reflexive about any prior professional relationships with participants. Being reflexive means reflecting on our own influence in a situation. There was regular reflection on how knowing and being known by participants might influence interviews and interpretation of stories. For example, after interviewing participants, I reflected on my perception of how they related to me. This revealed that I thought some related to me as a knowing listener to whom they could talk freely without having to explain terms and processes; others, as a trusted insider within education who was an ally in their troubles; and one, as a university-based outsider, unable to understand the priorities and realities of frontline practice. The trustworthiness of research is not mitigated by concealing potential influences but by being reflexively open and transparent about them. Nonetheless, the level of subjectivity within the practice of reflection gives rise to another ethical concern: credibility.

The credibility of research is closely tied to the claims made for the knowledge it generates (Connor, 2013). The claims made for this research are modest. It is not claimed that objective, generalisable fact has been found, but that insights which seem credible to other practice educators have been identified and shared.

The dependable quality of the research is rooted in transparent, traceable and documented decision-making. Its dependability is enhanced by transparent reflection and by sharing preliminary analysis and interpretation with other researchers. The research findings, implications and recommendations are confirmable because they are grounded in recorded stories (data) open to scrutiny in research supervision and audit.

Activity 1

What information do you need to give potential participants in your research that will enable them to feel confident that your research is ethical?

Review and evaluation of the research study

In this section of the chapter, practical issues arising from conducting narrative research are addressed, the extent to which the research design worked is discussed and there is reflection on what might be done differently were I to do this research again.

A significant practical issue in this study, and common in narrative research, was the problem of defining what a story is and then identifying stories within the transcribed interviews.

The definition adopted for stories in this research was that they were to be brief accounts of experience organised around characters, setting and plot (Riessman, 2004). A plot is the feature of a story that brings sequence and consequence, influencing how the storyteller organises events. The sequence of the story refers to the order of events: this event happened and then that event happened. When the storyteller states that what happens next is because of those initial events, consequence is revealed. Labov and Waletzky (1967) identified the following elements of naturally occurring stories:

- an *abstract* (gives notice that a story is about to be told)
- *an orientation* (the what, why, when, where and/or who of the story)
- *a complicating event*, (what happened)
- *a response or a resolution* (what then happened as a result; consequence)
- *an evaluation* (the 'so what?' of the story: its meaning to the teller)
- *a coda* (marking the end of that speaker's turn in conversation)

For example, 'I've had such a bad day (abstract). I was going to do an interview (orientation), but my car broke down and I didn't get to the interview (complicating event) and because of that the participant has withdrawn from the research (consequence/result). It's a real nuisance having to recruit another participant (evaluation). What a day (coda)!'

Activity 2

Ask two friends to tell you about a good day they have enjoyed recently. In their replies, see if they tell you any stories which follow the structure set out earlier.

Using these story elements, a purposeful search for stories in the transcripts of the interviews was made. However, boundaries between stories and their surrounding text were not easily demarcated. The process of identifying stories was iterative and creative rather than mechanistic. In one interview, a participant began a story but made a lengthy digression before returning to finish the story. This digression was removed from the research story. In another, a participant returned again and again to the same event, telling me more and more about it throughout the interview. All these were brought together into one research story. In dialogical narrative analysis, it is the stories, rather than whole interviews, that are the focus of analysis and interpretation. However, because the researcher's identification of stories is itself an analytical act, the stories analysed and interpreted in the research need to be recognised as re/presentations of those told by participants.

Having ensured that the research was conducted ethically and having overcome the practical difficulty of identifying stories, the research approach worked well. The purpose of the research had been to gain fresh insight into practice educators' perception of and positioning in practice education, and this was well achieved. Dialogical narrative analysis (Frank, 2010, 2012) of the abundant stories practice educators told led to an understanding of their role as boundary workers because they work in an overlapping space between practice and education. In this space, practice educators are committed equally to being educators and to being practitioners, although the boundary between the two is complex and creates conflict. At that boundary, they encountered threats to their professional judgement and to their decisions from senior personnel within their own practice settings and from personnel within the university. Interpretation of their stories offered insight into their boundary working skills and strategies, which were sometimes deployed collaboratively and cooperatively, and at other times oppressively and collusively. What was found to be at stake in their stories was their capacity to work boundaries collaboratively because of constraints imposed on them by people in dominant positions in placement agencies and universities. Overall, the research was successful in bringing attention to these matters, which were of concern to practice educators.

On reflection, if I were to do this research again, the main thing I would do differently is to start thinking sooner about what the stories meant collectively. The danger of stories is that we get caught up in them, and I was captivated by a few individual stories that I explored for far too long individually at the expense of understanding them in the context of other equally important stories. I spent so long thinking *about* stories instead of thinking *with* them that, for a while, I lost sight of the dialogue between stories that belongs at the heart of dialogical narrative analysis. I began to create a coherent interpretation of the stories only when I began exploring relations (patterns, themes, dissonances, similarities) between them as a whole.

This reflection concludes with my perceptions of the advantages and disadvantages of dialogical narrative analysis (see Figure 8.3).

Advantages of dialogical narrative analysis	*Disadvantages of dialogical narrative analysis*
People generally enjoy sharing their experiences and so gathering stories is relatively easy.	Defining and maintaining a researcher role in narrative research can be difficult because of the particularly conversation style of narrative interviews.
Rich qualitative data can be relatively easily gathered.	Deciding on what counts as a story and then retaining that definition when analysing transcripts is challenging.
The voice of participants is strongly present in rich storied data.	Some participants' stories shout louder than others, demanding to be heard. Heeding them can be to the detriment of more quietly spoken stories.
It offers a good means of bringing practice and research together.	Researchers who are also practitioners in the field, and known to be such by participants, need to find a comfortable position in which to straddle that boundary.

Figure 8.3 Advantages and disadvantages of dialogical narrative analysis

Relevance of this research to social care practice

There are clear links between the processes of research and the values of social care and healthcare practice. Research, like healthcare and social care practice, requires high standards of ethical conduct in terms of behaving honestly and with integrity, being respectful and upholding people's dignity, ensuring consent is voluntary and informed, maintaining confidentiality and being trustworthy. Researchers, healthcare practitioners and social care practitioners alike need to be skilled communicators, able to build rapport and effective relationships appropriate to their respective roles. They need to be able to conduct interviews in a cordial and ethical way, ask questions clearly and probe deeper respectfully. Furthermore, they all need to be able to keep truthful, accurate records.

A key finding of this research was that practice educators work at and across boundaries where different actors with different kinds of power exert their authority either collusively and oppressively or collaboratively and cooperatively. Key learning from this was that disputes can be better managed by using boundary working skills. This is relevant to social care and healthcare because both are practised at and across boundaries. These include boundaries between services (housing, criminal justice, children's services, youth services, adults' services, older people's services, healthcare, social care and education), between sectors (private, voluntary and statutory) and between geographical locations. Although there is a need to address factors creating barriers to collaboration and cooperation (Pereira, 2019), the research presented in this chapter draws attention to the importance of developing skills and values associated with being cooperative and collaborative when working at boundaries. Respect, trust and integrity were confirmed as essential because they create conditions in which differences of role, priorities, interests and accountabilities can be understood and negotiated. Tact and diplomacy were apparent in stories where disputes at boundaries were resolved collaboratively. A willingness to build coalitions and work as allies, rather than defensively assert jurisdiction, clearly supported cooperative boundary working. Boundary working skills are the bedrock of a collaborative, inter-agency way of working that can improve the lives of people with lived experience of social care and healthcare (Adams, 2005; Oliver 2013, Williams, 2011).

Link to the full research study

Murr, A (2020). *Working the boundaries: A dialogical narrative analysis of practice educators' stories.* EdD. Thesis, University of Wolverhampton. [online] Available at: https://wlv.openrepository.com/bitstream/handle/2436/623713/Murr_Phd_thesis_Redacted.pdf?sequence=1&isAllowed=y.

Further reading

Caddick, N., Phoenix, C. and Smith, B. (2015). Collective stories and well-being: Using a dialogical narrative approach to understand peer relationships among combat veterans experiencing post-traumatic stress disorder. *Journal of Health Psychology*, 20(3), pp. 286–299. https://doi.org/10.1177/1359105314566612.

Frank, A. (2010). *Letting stories breathe: A socio-narratology*. Chicago: The University of Chicago Press.

Patterson, W. (2008). Narrative of events: Labovian narrative analysis and its limitations. In: M. Andrews, C. Squire, and M. Tamboukou, eds., *Doing narrative research*. London: Sage, pp. 27–46.

Stone, C. (2016). The role of practice educators in initial and post qualifying social worker education. *Social Work Education*, 35(6), pp. 706–718.

References

Adams, R. (2005). Working within and across boundaries: Tensions and dilemmas. In: R. Adams, L. Dominelli, and M. Payne, eds., *Social work futures*. Basingstoke: Palgrave Macmillan, pp. 99–114.

Bolton, G. and Delderfield, R. (2018). *Reflective practice, writing and professional practice,* 5th ed. London: Sage.

Cohen, L., Manion, L. and Morrison, K. (2011). *Research methods in education.* Abingdon: Routledge.

Connor, S. (2013). *What's your problem? Making sense of social problems and the policy process.* Northwich: Critical Publishing.

Creswell, J. (2018). *Qualitative inquiry and research design: Choosing among five approaches,* 4th ed. London: Sage.

Domakin, A. (2014). Are we making the most of learning from the practice placement? *Social Work Education,* 33(6), pp. 718–730.

Frank, A. (2010). *Letting stories breathe: A socio-narratology.* Chicago: The University of Chicago Press.

Frank, A. (2012). Practicing dialogical narrative analysis. In: J.A. Holstein and J.F. Gubrium, eds., *Varieties of narrative analysis.* London: Sage, pp. 33–52.

Hancock, L. (2016). Introduction: Narrative, identity, and social movement activism. In: L. Hancock, ed., *Narratives of identity in social movements, conflicts and change: Research in social movements, conflicts and change,* Vol. 40. Bingley: Emerald Group Publishing Limited, pp. xi–xvii.

Jovchelovitch, S. and Bauer, M. (2000). *Narrative interviewing.* London: LSE Research Online. [online] Available at: http://eprints.lse.ac.uk/2633 [Accessed 30 Dec. 2020].

Labov, W. and Waletzky, J. (1967). Narrative analysis. In: J. Helm, ed., *Essays on the verbal and visual arts.* Seattle: University of Washington Press, pp. 12–44. [online] Available at: www.google.com/url?sa=t&rct=j&q=&esrc=s&source=web&cd=1&ved=2ahUKEwiJwYWenOLmAhURVRUIHX1pCawQFjAAegQIBRAC&url=http%3A%2F%2Fwww.ling.upenn.edu%2F~rnoyer%2Fcourses%2F103%2Fnarrative.pdf&usg=AOvVaw1jpBIhOSReQaT5WbO3Se2 [Accessed 13 Feb. 2021].

Oliver, C. (2013). Social workers as boundary spanners: Reframing our professional identity for interprofessional practice. *Social Work Education,* 32(6), pp. 773–784.

Pereira, M. (2019). Boundary-work that does not work: Social inequalities and the non-performativity of scientific boundary-work. *Science, Technology, & Human Values,* 44(2), pp. 338–365. doi: 10.1177/0162243918795043.

Riessman, C.K. (2004). Narrative analysis. In: M.S. Lewis-Beck, A. Bryman, and T. Futing Liao, eds., *Encyclopedia of social science research methods*. London: Sage, pp. 705–709.

Savin-Baden, M. and van Niekerk, L. (2007). Narrative inquiry: Theory and practice. *Journal of Geography in Higher Education*, 31(3), pp. 459–472.

Squire, C. (2008). From experience centred to socio-culturally-oriented approaches to narrative. In: M. Andrews, C. Squire, and M. Tamboukou, eds., *Doing narrative research*. London: Sage, pp. 47–71.

Williams, P. (2011). The life and times of the boundary spanner. *Journal of Integrated Care*, 19(3), pp. 26–33.

Woods, T. (2015). Practice educators' experiences of facilitating and assessing student values and ethics learning: Constructing dialogue. *Social Work Education*, 34(8), pp. 936–951.

9 An ethnographic approach to researching the communication of people with severe learning disabilities

Stephanie Brewster

Introduction

'Communication is at the heart of who we are as human beings' (Jagoe, no date) and the right to express opinions and communicate information is enshrined in Article 19 of the Universal Declaration of Human Rights. Communication is also the medium through which we exercise a wide range of other human rights such as participating in community, education and leisure. Most people with learning disabilities experience communication difficulties – some have little or no speech – and are therefore at risk of being unheard, excluded and marginalised. Without effective communication, these individuals cannot control their lives, build relationships and express their feelings, thoughts and needs.

This chapter discusses doctoral research conducted in small group homes for adults with severe learning disabilities. Such settings are part of a wider societal and political context in which people with disabilities are oppressed and devalued. Those with limited communication are further disadvantaged, and this research aimed to investigate how this is evident in the everyday interaction between residents and their care staff.

Recognising the ethical ideal that research about disability is conducted by disabled people themselves, there are nevertheless distinct methodological challenges and ethical issues entailed in people

DOI: 10.4324/9781003157724-9

with cognitive and communication impairments being involved in the research process. While striving to demonstrate an emancipatory ethos, the research encountered issues of capacity to consent to participate and a lack of tried and tested analytical tools that could accommodate the highly asymmetrical interaction between individuals with very limited communication skills and their much more articulate care staff. The research took an ethnographic approach in which rich qualitative data in the form of field notes, interviews with care staff and video recordings of 'real life' interaction were gathered over a long period spent in the 'field' (the natural social setting). This chapter makes a case for prolonged periods of engagement with individuals who may communicate in unconventional ways and the centrality of issues of power.

Background and outline of the research

This research stemmed from a personal wish to discover the reasons why so many adults with learning disabilities and limited or no verbal communication who were provided with communication aids (such as symbol boards and electronic devices) did not use them. This issue had long been recognised as widespread, and as a Speech and Language Therapist, the researcher had encountered many such situations. From this initial, vague motivation, the research questions emerged and became refined as the project progressed; the aim became to analyse the interaction between residents and staff in terms of power relations and to consider the differences in both power and communication skills between people with learning disabilities and their care staff (their main communication partners).

Research questions

1. To critically analyse the interaction between residents and staff in terms of power relations
2. To explore the hypothesis that power relations contribute to a lack of communication aid use

There is a variety of terminologies used to label research in which people with disabilities have been involved to various extents. Riddell, Baron and Wilson (2001) refer to this collectively as the 'democratic disability research paradigm'. Such research is collaborative, self-aware and critical. It values the contribution of those who need help to express their views, values difference and avoids recreating the traditional hierarchy within societies as a whole, as well as within the research context. This research project did not aim for objectivity and neutrality, but rather it adopted an openly ideological stance regarding the position of people with severe learning disabilities in society. It has been argued that ethnographic research should not only aim to understand the world but also to change it; in other words, it should be 'emancipatory', the goal being to contribute to the freedom and empowerment of marginalised or disadvantaged people (in this case those with learning disabilities) in an equal and just society.

Ethnography is an approach to qualitative research which involves participating in people's lives over a long period of time (Hammersley and Atkinson, 2007, p. 3), gathering a variety of data through, for example observing what happens and asking questions. In other words, everyday contexts are studied in depth in a naturalistic or unstructured way. A small number of settings are usually selected. Analysis of these predominantly verbal data entails 'interpretation of the meanings, functions, and consequences of human actions and institutional practices' (Hammersley and Atkinson, 2007, p. 3). It takes an exploratory orientation in which initially broad areas of interest become gradually more refined, and specific research questions emerge. This emergent quality, characteristic of ethnography, is evident in the project being discussed here.

Although much has been written about the ethical issue of securing consent to participate in research, it could be argued that the systematic exclusion of people such as those with severe learning disabilities who are not readily able to demonstrate capacity to consent is of equal or even greater concern. As Dee-Price et al. (2021) also point out, research findings rarely capture the first-person insights of people with complex communication access needs.

Nevertheless, we need to be honest about the feasibility of people with severe learning disabilities participating in or controlling their own research. Considerable challenges arise when attempting to conduct emancipatory research with people with severe learning disabilities. The very nature of learning disability means that those experiencing it are unlikely to have the intellectual skills necessary for participation in research in conventional ways, and many will have internalised the power relationships which emancipatory research seeks to challenge. The researcher agrees with Clegg, who says 'I struggle to understand why anyone imagines they could obtain informed consent to, say, research participation from a multiply disabled adult with a developmental age of 3 months' (Clegg, 2003, p. 4). However, some methodological progress is being made; Dee-Price et al. (2021) for example discuss their development and testing of new methods of data collection that could improve access to research for people with complex communication access needs. The research being discussed in this chapter also concerns people who are, at least to an extent, unable to 'articulate and reflect upon their experiences' (Klotz, 2004, p. 101). Klotz (2004) makes a case for approaches which do not rely on eliciting data from people with learning disabilities but which place interaction and relationships centrally in naturalistic contextual observations. Ethnography is therefore a valuable approach, since people's behaviour is considered within its natural context; it allows the time needed to get to know them well, to maximise their communication and participation in the research. And although the researcher cannot claim to have undertaken emancipatory research, this ethos influenced all stages of the research.

Accessing settings, sampling and recruiting participants

'Fieldwork' refers to research in which data is gathered in naturally occurring social settings. The process of negotiating access to fieldwork sites (residential homes, in this case) was implicit in every visit to the sites, but it was most explicit early in the programme of fieldwork. As soon as ethical approval from the NHS was received, the directorate manager of social care homes was approached and provided contact details of the managers of several care homes. Each home manager handled the researcher's approach differently and included invitations to staff meetings, informal visits and an interview; on each occasion, information sheets about the research were supplied. Their appreciation of the topic as an important area in need of investigation may have been influential in the positive and enthusiastic response all managers gave to the proposed research.

Five small residential homes for adults with learning disabilities were selected, being judged as fairly typical of their type. Within each setting, further sampling occurred in terms of decisions about 'where to observe and when, who to talk to and what to ask, as well as about what to record and show' (Hammersley and Atkinson, 2007, p. 35). Four individual residents who could communicate intentionally, verbally and/or non-verbally and a small number of staff were selected for in-depth study.

Methods of data collection

Data was collected over the course of a year, through weekly visits to the homes; initially, the methods used were observations and interviews with staff, which were later supplemented with videos of resident–staff interactions.

Participant observation

Handwritten notes were taken while in the field, then typed in more detail immediately afterwards and meticulously organised and archived. Field notes were initially very broad but gradually narrowed in focus and became more selective over time; the behaviour and interaction of people were the main research interest. Adopting the role of 'observer-as-participant' (Cohen, Manion and Morrison, 2011, p. 457) enabled the researcher to be unobtrusive at times, joining in with activities at others. Field notes served two functions: to support the development of a clear focus for the research and as background information to enhance the interpretation of video data.

Interviewing staff

Interviews tended to be informal spontaneous conversations, which blurred into participant observation (Hammersley and Atkinson, 2007); this was beneficial, as rapport had already been established between the researcher and the staff member, prior to conducting interviews. Also, conducting interviews within their familiar environment helped participating staff relax and fitted into their work schedule. Interviews were unstructured, as is usual in ethnographic research; they were an important source of data, providing staff members' perspectives on their interaction with residents.

Video recording of resident–staff interactions

After a period of fieldwork, when trust and rapport had been established, naturally occurring interactions between staff and residents were video recorded; these can be described as unsolicited data (Hammersley and Atkinson, 2007) in contrast to the (solicited) interviews with staff. Re-watching the video clips enabled careful analysis of interactions, including both verbal and non-verbal (multi-modal) aspects of interaction.

Transcription of audio recordings of staff interviews and videos of interactions with residents, combined with contextual information from field notes, constituted the data set.

It is important to point out that such qualitative data is open to a range of interpretations; therefore, the validity of naturalistic qualitative research findings can be called into question. Rigour and confidence rather than certainty or objectivity (Cohen, Manion and Morrison, 2011, p. 181) are the aims. The prolonged engagement in the field, coupled with the triangulation of multiple methods of data collection, contributes to the credibility of the research (Cohen, Manion and Morrison, 2011). A certain amount of member checking or respondent validation (Hammersley and Atkinson, 2007) also supported the authenticity of the data; this occurred through the sharing of emerging findings and conclusions with (staff) participants – these would then be discussed further and elaborated or modified.

The processes of analysis and interpretation of data necessarily merged together, as it commonly does in qualitative research. The rich data set combined fine-grained detail with the broad social context in which interactions occurred. Discourse analysis was used: 'discourse analysis examines how meaning is constructed through texts. . . . It focuses on issues of power, domination and reproduction of power in texts and conversations, language in social contexts and interactions' (Cohen, Manion and Morrison, 2011, pp. 574–575). In this project, field notes, interview transcripts and transcripts of multi-modal interactions were all forms of 'text'. Given the subjective nature of this process, it was important for the researcher's possible biases to be made transparent; hence, at the outset the disempowerment of people with learning disabilities in society in general and within research was discussed. A number of key themes arose from the data and these were presented in the research report and illustrated with small passages of transcription to illuminate the discussion.

Key findings

Themes that emerged from the data in response to the aims of the research included turn-taking and topic control in interaction, politeness and the use of 'test questions' by staff (questions staff ask residents to which they know the answer; for example, 'What happened yesterday?'). In many respects, much of the staff–resident interactions resembled that between adults and children; but it was also evident that the residents were not entirely powerless in interaction. Nevertheless, staff were adept at controlling aspects of day-to-day interaction, at least partly in order to facilitate residents' participation in it. In the long term though, this significantly constrained the interaction, and residents did not have opportunities to develop more sophisticated communication skills or to express themselves more freely.

Ethical issues

Ethical issues are of central concern in any research, but nowhere is this more the case than among people with limited communication skills and intellectual ability. The British Psychological Society (BPS, 2018) code of ethics and conduct identifies four ethical principles, the first of which, 'Respect for the dignity of persons and peoples' was paramount throughout. The following discussion concentrates on the pragmatic issue of informed consent.

Decisions about an individual's capacity to make a decision on whether to participate in research depends on them being deemed able to do so free from coercion and it being based on an understanding of the research, its risks and benefits. A label of learning disabilities (or any other label) cannot be used to assume they lack capacity. However, for most people with severe learning disabilities their ability to understand information, reach a decision and communicate it will be impaired, and so they will not be regarded as having capacity. This needs to be balanced with the need to ensure they are not excluded (Cameron and Murphy, 2006, p. 118), and researchers are required to take all practicable steps to support a person to make a decision (BPS, 2020). For this research, the NHS ethics committee required information for residents to be provided in alternative 'easy read' formats (even though none of the residents were considered by their care staff to be able to understand either text or symbols, revealing the committee's lack of insight into the group of people being potentially included). Nevertheless, the information leaflets created followed Mencap's (2002) Guidelines for Accessible Writing and proved useful for other participants, such as care staff. Cameron and Murphy (2006) remind us of the importance of providing accessible and understandable information using supports such as symbols, simple language, bullet points and repetition of information.

It remained the case though, that 'When it comes to ideas which are more complex there is unlikely to be a substitute for working alongside people who know the individual well and can draw on the experience of what works with him or her' (Cameron and Murphy, 2006. p. 116). Indeed, for this research, none of the residents was able to give explicit voluntary informed consent. In line with the BPS guidance (2020), wider consultation was important: the care home managers, key workers and family members were the 'consultees' involved in deciding whether the residents could be considered happy to participate. The decision was always taken after several visits, and it had become clear to carers that the resident was comfortable with the researcher's presence. Those who knew the resident well were asked to identify what signals might indicate that the resident was not happy with the researcher's presence. It was important to give assurances about the confidentiality of data, especially video footage, about which there was most sensitivity.

Although the risks of being involved in the research were very low, with no invasive procedures, the use of video in particular made it potentially 'intrusive' (BPS, 2020). All staff agreed to be interviewed informally and to be observed, but the majority refused consent for video recordings to be made of them, commenting on their embarrassment and self-consciousness. The selective granting of consent from staff resulted in significant curtailment of the amount and nature of data collected. Researchers also need to be sensitive to the possibility of opening up unanticipated areas of discussion (Cameron and Murphy, 2006), a risk in this research that was greater for staff than for residents. It is widely recognised that consent should be regarded as an ongoing process, not just a one-off event at the outset of research. Relationships between participants and myself were of greater value than merely following procedures, when it came to ensuring ethical conduct.

Activity 1

Ethical guidance and standards are constantly changing. Identify the professional body and current guidelines relevant to your research. How will you apply these ethical guidelines to all the stages of your project: your overall research design, your methodology, data collection and analysis and the dissemination of your findings?

Practical issues in undertaking this research approach

Limitations in the extent to which the learning-disabled participants were involved in shaping the project have already been discussed; inevitably, there were other practical concerns such as those arising from the compromise between breadth and depth. Data collection was conducted at five homes in all; while this may strengthen the case for some generalisation of conclusions, it resulted in field relationships of insufficient depth for participation in the project to have any transformatory effect. The initial hope had been for participation to facilitate the personal development of staff in terms of their interaction with residents. But this underestimated how difficult this might be to achieve: challenging beliefs and assumptions and changing habits can be an uncomfortable and long process.

Another major area of practical concern was the video recording and transcription of data. The use of video is a powerful way to capture the idiosyncratic and often fleeting modes of communication used by people with severe learning disabilities, although it is in no way objective: it too is open to interpretation. The same point may be made about transcription of video footage; when meanings may be highly ambiguous, care needs to be taken to be open about the nature of the interpretative process carried out by the researcher and (more powerful) others such as family members and carers.

Transcription is time-consuming (Hammersley and Atkinson, 2007), taking at least five times as long as the duration of the recording to transcribe into written text, (although voice recognition software is improving all the time and can make the process much less arduous). Interviews with staff were transcribed in full, usually from audiotape using widely used orthographic transcription conventions, to capture only the words that were said.

However, much more fine-grained transcription was conducted on the video footage of interaction involving residents, which aimed to represent the non-verbal nature of much of this interaction. It took well over an hour to transcribe a minute of interaction in this way, so careful selection was necessary: the aim was to achieve a sample of transcribed data that was broadly representative of all of the data in terms of participants and activities or settings. No transcription provides a complete record of interaction; so, strategic decisions had to be made about what to transcribe and what details to include, based on the aims of the research.

There were two main challenges in transcribing this multi-modal interaction. First, how to convey meaning: a good knowledge of the context and the individual are required for intended meaning to be interpreted correctly and use of field notes helped in interpreting the interactions. Second, how to present the transcription in such a way as to avoid inadvertently privileging spoken utterances over non-verbal communication and giving prominence to the speaking partner over the less verbal individual. Therefore, the residents' interaction was placed to the left of the page and non-verbal behaviours to the left of verbal or vocal information. Presenting one line of transcription per second enabled the reader to get a sense of pace of the interaction and gave information about relative times that each participant held the floor – an aspect which could be relevant to the analysis of power relations (see Figure 9.1).

Once transcriptions were complete, they and field notes underwent several processes of analysis. First they were split into segments, each consisting of several lines of text; these were identified by date and location. Each segment was then given one or more codes that related to the aims of the research, for example 'choice', 'fun/banter', 'care needs' 'control'. A long list of codes were generated, and these were gradually refined and grouped into themes or categories. With the help of a database, segments of data could be retrieved by code; then by placing them alongside each other it was possible to explore patterns in the data such as which codes tended to occur together and how frequently. This enabled analysis to work upwards from the data but also to work in a downward direction from theory and from the research questions. Cohen, Manion and Morrison (2007) provide a useful overview of the many ways in which qualitative data can be analysed and discuss the inevitable risk of researcher subjectivity that arises.

Venue: Number 32
Date: 27.04.04
Setting: kitchen, following cookery session
Participants: resident Sarah; staff Sue; researcher behind camera.
Duration: 33 seconds
Selection criteria: coded as 'requesting'

Key:
→ looks towards . . .
← looks away
▶ points towards
(n) unintelligible speech, (number of syllables)

Time (secs)	*Resident: non-verbal*	*Resident: verbal/vocal*	*Staff: non-verbal*	*Staff: verbal*
1.	→ Sue	I'm wet	Back to camera, wiping crumbs off S's tray and footstool	
2.				You're wet?
3.		umm		
4.				You sure you're wet

Figure 9.1 An example of multi-modal transcription involving a resident with some speech

Evaluation, dissemination, impact and final reflections

A common criticism of ethnographic research is the lack of real-world impact. Research impact is discussed extensively nowadays, with many research projects explicitly setting out how their research will bring about real-world benefits. In fully emancipatory research, feedback of research outcomes to participants and wider dissemination is a requirement, but more than this is required to bring about change. In hindsight, the researcher recognised that the focus was too narrowly on the dissemination of findings to the participants and other stakeholders. But even this was, unfortunately, very challenging. The nature of the findings entailed abstract theorising of concepts which were out of the reach of many of those with learning disabilities. To an extent the same could be said for the staff, whose generally practical orientation to their work allowed little space for reflection of a more theoretical or abstract nature. At a pragmatic level, the prolonged duration of the project spanned considerable staff turnover and it proved difficult to sustain relationships with them through the final dissemination phase of the research. Dissemination to the wider research community took the form of several publications and presentations – a time-consuming phase of research that required considerable forward planning and consideration.

For the residents in this research, care staff provided most, if not all of their social contact. The relationships between them, in which both practical assistance and also companionship are important, are of huge significance to the quality of life of the residents. Day-to-day interaction can enhance empowerment and choice in residents' lives, but it can also disempower and control them; this research provided evidence of both occurring in a fluid dynamic imperceptible to the participants.

People with learning disabilities are amongst the most disempowered in our society, and policies and services provided to them have often been accused of reinforcing this situation. Meaningful participation in decisions about their own lives is a particular challenge for people with the most severe learning disabilities: choice and control are unavailable when there is no communication.

Research on communication has so far concentrated its attention on language while failing to address issues of power. And yet this research demonstrates that residential care homes like these often reflect, to an extent, societal conditions of oppression of people with disabilities. Training for staff in interaction techniques should also address staff values and attitudes and raise awareness of the power relations within interaction.

Only by ensuring the inclusion of people with communication impairments in research can we get a better understanding of the challenges they face in their day-to-day lives (Dee-Price et al., 2021). Through communication, individuals exercise choice and control over their lives, build relationships and express themselves. Communication is a human right.

Activity 2

All research proposals must be realistic. Starting with your research idea or topic, begin considering the practical details including:

- What settings will be your research sites? How many participants do you hope to recruit? What data collection methods will you use? What are the ethical issues?
- Make a list of the possible barriers or limitations you may encounter in conducting your research.
- Note down how you will address any challenges that arise.

Link to the full research study

Brewster, S. Asymmetries of power and competence and implications for AAC: interaction between adults with severe learning disabilities and their care staff.

Unpublished EdD thesis, University of Birmingham http://etheses.bham.ac.uk/63/

Further reading

Brewster, S. (2013). Saying the 'F word . . . in the nicest possible way': Augmentative communication and discourses of disability. *Disability & Socety*, 28(1), pp. 125–128. doi: 10.1080/09687599.2012.736672.

Williams, V. (2011). *Disability and discourse: Analysing inclusive conversation with people with intellectual disabilities*. West Sussex: Wiley Blackwell.

References

British Psychological Society. (2018). *Code of ethics and conduct*. [online] Available at: www.bps.org.uk/sites/www.bps.org.uk/files/Policy/Policy%20-%20Files/BPS%20Code%20of%20Ethics%20

and%20Conduct%20%28Updated%20July%202018%29.pdf [Accessed 20 Feb. 2021].

British Psychological Society. (2020). *Conducting research with people not having the capacity to consent to their participation: A practical guide for researchers.* [online] Available at: www.bps.org.uk/sites/www.bps.org.uk/files/Policy/Policy%20-%20Files/Conducting%20research%20with%20people%20not%20having%20the%20capacity%20to%20consent.pdf [Accessed 20 Feb. 2021].

Cameron, L. and Murphy, J. (2006). Obtaining consent to participate in research: The issues involved in including people with a range of learning and communication disabilities. *British Journal of Learning Disabilities*, 35(2), pp. 113–120.

Clegg, J. (2003). The ideal proxy informant. *Ethics and Intellectual Disability*, 7(2), pp. 1 and 4–5.

Cohen, L., Manion, L. and Morrison, K. (2007). *Research methods in education.* London: Routledge.

Cohen, L, Manion, L. and Morrison, K. (2011). *Research methods in education*, 7th ed. London: Routledge.

Dee-Price, B-J M., Hallahan, L., Nelson Bryen, D. and Watson, J.M. (2021). Every voice counts: Exploring communication accessible research methods. *Disability & Society*, 36(2), pp. 240–264. doi: 10.1080/09687599.2020.1715924.

Hammersley, M. and Atkinson, P. (2007). *Ethnography: Principles in practice*, 3rd ed. Routledge.

Jagoe, C. (no date). *Why is communication a basic human right?* [online] Available at: https://internationalcommunicationproject.com/profile/communication-basic-human-right/ [Accessed 5 May 2021].

Klotz, J. (2004). Sociocultural study of intellectual disability: Moving beyond labelling and social constructionist perspectives. *British Journal of Learning Disabilities*, 32(2), pp. 93–104.

Mencap. (2002). *Making myself clear.* [online] Available at: www.accessibleinfo.co.uk/pdfs/Making-Myself-Clear.pdf [Accessed 20 Feb. 2021].

Riddell, S, Baron, S. and Wilson, A. (2001). *The learning society and people with learning difficulties.* Bristol: The Polity Press.

10 Exploring perceptions of professional expertise within a health and social care context

Theresa Kinnersley

Introduction

The focus of this book is to increase the accessibility of research as a concept to those working within health and social care contexts. This chapter serves to support this aim and demonstrate how 'the questions we ask do matter' (Charmaz, 2017, p. 34). Whilst deciding upon the research topic, or area of interest is important, it is also worth taking time to really consider what it is you want to find out; what do you want to know that you do not know already . . . and what difference might it make within the practice-based, professional context?

The main focus of this chapter is upon enabling the reader to gain insight into a mixed methods data collection method as a novel means of exploration and discovery. Research should be exciting, and the aim of this chapter is to demonstrate how the questions we ask can influence the development and impact of the research study itself. This chapter is based upon the reflections on a specific research study that was completed in 2019, the focus of which was to increase awareness and access to professional development.

The focus for the particular research study in question was upon the construction of a tool to assist professionals reflect upon and learn from their personal and professional experiences. The hope was that if a tool could assist this process, then the professionals in question could be supported to develop a level of expertise, with benefit both

DOI: 10.4324/9781003157724-10

to themselves and those they were working with. Expertise as a concept has gained in significance since the 1950s, however, it is still an area that is poorly researched. Whilst there is no certainty that reflection enables the development of expertise, there is an awareness that expertise is both valuable and worthy of investment (King et al., 2007).

The particular research study in question has at its centre a profession known as Conductive Education (CE). Conductive Education is a holistic, person-centred approach to working with children and adults with neuromotor disorders such as cerebral palsy, stroke and Parkinson's (Szogeczki, 2017). The conductor as the professional who delivers this person-centred programme of learning within Statutory and Third Sector health and education provisions has gained a BA in CE and Qualified Conductor Status (QCS). Whilst the reader may have never heard of CE, or come into contact with a conductor, the research process discussed here can be considered applicable to those working in other person-centred professions, such as nursing, social care and education (Hattie, 2003; Kinchin, Cabot and Hay, 2008). All of those working within these contexts come into contact with individuals and their families who need support. As such these professionals need not only to acquire knowledge and skill but also the motivation to continue making a positive impact upon the individuals they are caring for and working with.

The Latin adjective 'expertus' means 'to have tried' or 'to have experienced' (Eraut, 2005, p. 173) and is considered to be the root word from which both experience and expertise have developed (Germain and Ruiz, 2009). Expertise is dependent upon experience; however, it is not synonymous with it (Wainwright et al., 2011). It is therefore possible to see the two as related but uniquely different. Expertise is neither domain-, role- or position-specific (Germain and Tejeda, 2012). Commonality amongst person-centred professions suggests that expert practice includes a mix of knowledge, skill and personal application (Brody and Hadar, 2015). Few research studies exist in which perceptions of expertise are explored (Germain and Ruiz, 2009), however, expertise is valued as a significant aspect of professional development. It was therefore considered relevant to consider the ways in which expert practice is perceived within CE and the factors that may influence the construction of these perceptions. With this in mind, the following research questions were determined.

Research questions

1. How do conductors construct their perception of professional expertise?
2. What are the common priorities associated with the professional expertise of the conductor?
3. Is it possible to measure professional expertise?
4. Can a measure of professional expertise be used to facilitate professional development?

The first thing to consider was how to answer these research questions. Returning to Charmaz's (2017) awareness of the significance of the question, consideration was given to the choice of underpinning research methodology and the data collection methods.

Conductive education has an underpinning theoretical basis which is both constructivist and constructionist in nature (Grundtvig, 2012). Both constructionism and constructivism involve social interaction (Guba, 1990); whilst constructionism impacts ideas as a consequence of conversation and social interaction, constructivism is considered a biological, cognitive process of individual meaning making (Wink and Wink, 2004). Within the research study, it was this individual process of 'meaning making' that was considered significant.

Personal construct theory

Personal construct theory (PCT), the work of George Kelly (1963) sits within the constructivist paradigm (Kuipers and Grice, 2009) and was chosen as the underpinning research methodology. PCT creates opportunity to consider how individuals construct their unique perception of reality in specific contexts, for example one person's experiences of the COVID-19 pandemic will be similar to but not the same as another's. Within the context of the research, it was the professional's perceptions of expertise that were important to determine. . . . for example what made them think person A was an expert, but person B was not?

As a process of articulated 'meaning-making', construing is described as a holistic combination of thought, action and cognition (Kelly, 1963; Marsden and Littler, 2000). Language is used to determine in explicit terms the meaning that a specific event or role has to that individual by definition of what it means to them. The meanings attached to these events are referred to as constructs. Constructs are defined as bipolar, hierarchical and interconnected (Raskin, 2002). For example, if you were asked to define what a healthy diet was, you might articulate this as plant-based food. In contrast, you might describe those who ate meat as eating unhealthily. In a wider context, you might define yourself as ethical because you eat a plant-based diet, source clothes and food locally and recycle as much as possible. In contrast, you might define someone who eats meat, buys what they want regardless of where it came from and throws unwanted food and clothes in the bin as behaving in an 'unethical' manner. One of your peers however may argue the complete opposite. From this, it can be perceived that constructs are personal to the individual and reflect not only behaviours but the meanings attached to these behaviours; there are no 'rights or wrongs', as the significance is the individual's alone.

Activity 1

Write down one word that to you describes.

1. A face-to-face lecture
2. An online lecture
3. An online social event

(Remember these are YOUR perceptions. There are no 'rights' or 'wrongs'– perceptions are unique to you!) Then write down the opposite of these word. . . . Ask the same of a peer!

Congratulations, you have now constructed a bipolar construct pair!

Now, reflect upon the ways in which your perceptions are similar to those of your peers, but also different. Your answers give you an insight into what is important to each of you as unique individuals. You may not have known this prior to the exercise. For example, if you had just talked to your friends about lectures you may have focused only on one aspect of them, but by considering both the similarities and the differences you have new insights. This application serves to demonstrate the potential that PCT has to enable the 'tacit', or hidden, to be made explicit (Jankowicz, 2004).

Research method: the repertory grid technique

Personal construct theory is however just a theory. In order to apply this theory in practice, a data collection tool is required. The repertory grid technique (RGT) considered useful in exploratory studies where there is little prior research links directly to PCT as a data collection method. The RGT likened to a structured interview (Steed and McDonnell, 2012) can be utilised within a range of therapeutic, professional and research contexts (Pavlovic, 2011). As an adaptable mixed methods tool, the RGT fits well in health and social care research where quantitative data alone often proves insufficient to achieve the depth of study required (Darawsheh, 2014). The flexibility of the RGT makes it both appealing and vulnerable, as possibilities for its use are numerous. In the research study, the RGT was chosen for its potential to enable understanding of expertise beyond the predictable (Ralley et al., 2009). Whilst the RGT may be adapted to a range of contexts, all possibilities involve consideration of three main factors. With reference to the aforementioned application, we will consider each of these in turn and generate a repertory grid together.

Elements

The first of these three factors relate to the elements. The repertory grid is a matrix in which the elements form the columns. Rather than describe behaviours or objects, elements relate to people, events or activities (Jankowicz, 2004). You have already had experience of elements as can be seen in Table 10.1 in which the elements are inserted; 'face to face lectures', 'online lectures' and 'online social events'.

The RGT becomes a powerful tool for discovery by enabling the researcher to ask questions in relation to each of the elements. In the aforementioned application, you wrote words to reflect what each of these elements meant to you. You then wrote the opposite of these words.

Now you will insert these words into Table 10.2. Take each of the pair of words from the application and insert the first word from each pair in the 'first word' section and the second word in the 'second word' section. You have now inserted your three bipolar construct pairs into the grid. An example has been included to demonstrate.

Table 10.1 The grid structure with elements

Elements	*1*	*2*	*3*
	Face-to-face lectures	**Online lectures**	**Online social events**

Table 10.2 Grid example with elements and space for your own bipolar construct pairs (examples will be referred to later)

		Element 1	*Element 2*	*Element 3*		
	First word	**Face-to-face lectures**	**Online lectures**	**Online social events**	**Second word**	
Construct pair 1 Engaging						Construct pair 1 Isolating
Construct pair 2						Construct pair 2
Construct pair 3						Construct pair 3

Construct elicitation

As can be seen in Table 10.2, the construct pairs form rows (Steed and McDonnell, 2012). In this way it can be seen how the elements and construct pairs together help form the grid structure. From this example you now have experience of constructs as bipolar in nature. The pairs of words you have inserted create an understanding of what the elements mean to you but also what they do not mean. If you compare your bipolar construct pairs with your peer's you may see that your insights are similar but not exactly the same. Bipolar construct pairs give insight into what something means, and in contrast, what it does not mean to the individual in question.

The element–construct relationship

Once construct pairs have been articulated and inserted to the RGT, the next step is to numerically define the relationship between the elements and the constructs. By completing this part of the grid, you are able to demonstrate the mixed methods nature of the RGT. The construct pairs create opportunity to apply subjective interpretation of the data, whilst the numerical rating creates a more objective comprehension of perception. For this final stage of the RGT, go to Table 10.3 and consider each of the elements in turn. Now ask yourself, how 'similar' or 'different' each of the elements are to either of the words in each construct pair and 'rate' them accordingly. In the example (Table 10.3), the words Engaging and Isolating have been inserted, with corresponding numbers, for example face-to-face lectures are perceived to be more engaging than isolating and so are scored higher than online lectures which are perceived to be more isolating than engaging, and so are scored lower. By completing these stages, you have been able to utilise both PCT and the RGT to determine your perceptions in a unique manner. Whilst this is a simplification of the method, it perhaps expands opportunities for exploration of the individual, and what is important to them, as similar, but different to others.

Table 10.3 With example of scoring system. There is space to insert your own construct pairs and corresponding scoring

		Element 1	*Element 2*	*Element 3*		
	First word/ similar 3	**Face-to-face lectures**	**Online lectures**	**Online social event s**	**Second word/ different 1**	
Construct pair 1 Engaging		3	1	2		Construct pair 1 Isolating
Construct pair 2						Construct pair 2
Construct pair 3						Construct pair 3

Ethical issues

With reference to the British Psychological Society code of ethics and conduct (BPS, 2019) consideration was given to the application of respectful, confidential and professional research. Part-time and qualitative researchers who may more frequently be part of the group under investigation have to consider their status as 'insider-researchers' (Moore, 2012; Unluer, 2012). Perceived to be a mixed blessing (Mercer, 2007), there is potential to increase acceptance and award a degree of trust and connectedness simply because of the shared experiences. There is however also greater opportunity to exploit the relationship (Sutcliffe, Linfield and Geldart, 2012). I considered myself to be an insider-researcher; I was known to research participants but not working with them directly (Unluer, 2012). The reflexive nature of the insider-researcher fits well within a constructivist paradigm in which the researcher is explicitly 'present' within the study (Charmaz, 2006). This means it is possible to recognise and mitigate biases and perceptions that will influence how the study develops. This explicit presence serves to strengthen, rather than weaken the study. With an aim to determine perceptions there was less concern regarding a conflict of interest, however, to increase confidence, it was explicitly stated that findings would not be relayed directly to management (Mercer, 2007). Whilst my aim was to stay true to the data (Jankowicz, 2004), being an insider-researcher meant that in the write-up all identifying data was removed.

Sample and recruitment

Representing around one fifth of the conductors working in the UK, 20 conductors, considered an appropriate number of participants, were recruited to the study (Smith, 2000). Individual conductors were contacted via a 'gatekeeper', and where relevant, directly in person. Demographic information was collected prior to each interview. This data was correlated with each interview; however, the consent form was stored separately. Conductors were assured prior to interview of their right to withdraw and that all data was anonymous, confidential and stored securely.

Review and evaluation of the study – practical issues

Research takes time. Involving others in your work means that you have to allow for the unexpected, for conversations to over-run and for planning, piloting, reading, analysing and synthesising. Application of PCT in the form of the RGT is no exception, however, if it is the tacit, less tangible aspects that you are interested in, then this is a feasible and exciting approach.

Pilot the grid. Don't be tempted to make the grid too large, consider a smaller more focused grid to begin with. Ensure that you use elements that relate to people, events or activities and not emotions or behaviours. Be sure to include 'self' as an element, otherwise, you have lost a key part of the methodology (see application later). The RGT is a potential tool for change, and whilst it was not used for this purpose, you might consider it suitable to record change in perception following training or specific treatment interventions.

The aim was to explore the nature of, and gain insight into, the ways and means by which conductor's perceptions of expertise were both idiosyncratic, and similar, or different to others within the profession. The software programme, Idiogrid (www.idiogrid.com/), and application of Principal Component Analysis enabled synthesis of the data with respect to both individual and generic realities as a basis for further constructivist thematic analysis (Charmaz, 2006).

Key findings

1. Expertise is perceived to be a '*whole-istic*' combination of belief, personality, knowledge and skill (Figure 10.1).
2. Synthesis of findings suggests that conductors transit along a journey from novice to expert; however, whilst some are able to continue developing, others appear to become 'stuck' in position. In part, this journey is influenced by the experiences within the professional environment. This includes the presence or absence of a positive and supportive working environment, for example a cohesive peer group and shared values.
3. The acceptance and recognition of role models as a significant aspect of the professional environment is considered important if expertise is to be perceived as achievable.
4. Expertise can only develop as a consequence of experience and an ability to use experience to analyse, reflect and widen understanding of 'self' within the wider professional context (Benner (1984); Dreyfus and Dreyfus, 1986). The professional environment, in particular the impact of positive interpersonal relationships at all levels, is a significant factor in enabling experiential, tacit learning to develop, in particular the ability to expand perceptions of expertise as 'whole-istic'.
5. It is possible to construct a research study in which all aspects connect: a solution to the defined 'problem' can be elicited if consideration is given to both the theory and the practical application of that theory.

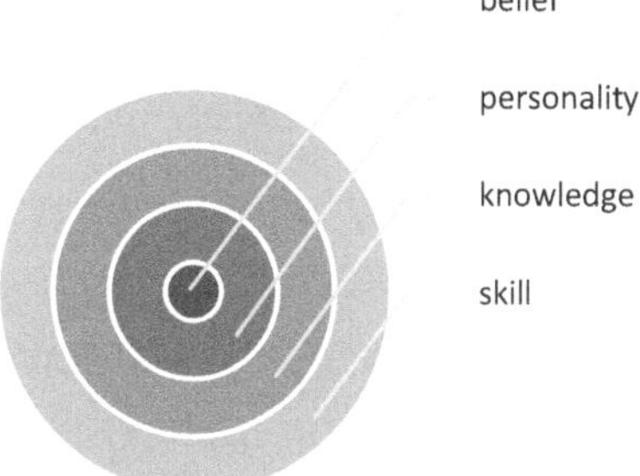

Figure 10.1

6. Is it possible to measure professional expertise?

   There currently exists no definition of expertise within CE, and the findings of this study do not generate a validated definition; however, it is possible to create a common perception of expertise (see Figure 10.1) as the basis from which a self-reflective measurement tool can be constructed with potential to assist all conductors to develop further.

7. Can a measure of professional expertise be used to facilitate professional development?

   The Values in Action (VIA) questionnaire was adapted to fit the professional context (Peterson and Seligman, 2004; McGovern and Miller, 2008). Self-actualisation as a process in which free will and potential combine to create the highest professionalism sits well within a positive psychology, strengths-based approach to professional development (Kamath and Ashok, 2015; Niemiec, 2018). Rather than categorise practitioners as novice, experienced or expert, the self-assessment measurement tool generated from the study serves to encourage development towards a perceived best practice, the priorities of which are determined by the individual.

Reflection and learning from the process – advantages and disadvantages of the approach

Key points learnt:

- It is possible to investigate and explore perceptions of less tangible aspects of life. PCT is one methodology that supports the articulation of the tacit making it explicit.
- The RGT, by utilising both quantitative and qualitative data, enables insight into both individual and generic perceptions of expertise.

Advantages and application to practice

As a subjective mapping tool, the RGT facilitates articulation of internal perceptual links and enables comprehension of individual construing. By generating both qualitative meaning and quantitative objectivity in the form of constructs and numerical ratings, the RGT has potential to generate understanding in a way that other methods do not so easily facilitate (Steed and McDonnell, 2012). In relation to the research study, it was not the actions of the expert that were explored but rather conductor's perceptions of the actions and behaviours they perceived as expert.

Disadvantages

It is possible to analyse data both quantitatively and qualitatively; however, familiarity with the data analysis methods takes time. This is both an advantage; triangulation of meaning and a disadvantage in that both numerical and thematic analysis are required. However, when both sources of data are analysed, a robust synthesis is possible.

Research dissemination

The findings of the study were disseminated to conductors via a range of sources; professional conferences – both national and international; as an article in the *Conductive College Journal* and as input to training and postgraduate education.

Application/relevance to the health and social care context

Consideration of expertise as a concept, and as an achievable goal for all in any profession, surely has a role to play in the development of that profession and the care given to service users. The findings of the first phase of the study led to the development of a self-assessment CPD tool. This tool, whilst not a validated measure of expertise, has potential to assist professional development at both individual and strategic levels.

Activity 1

1. The elements in the RGT relate to people, events or activities. Think of yourself in your professional role. Using the method outlined earlier, personalise the elements (suggested ideas have been inserted) and then generate bipolar construct pairs to represent each of them. In turn, insert each of the pairs of words into the grid and then score each of the elements against each of the construct pairs.
2. Well done. You have applied your learning to the professional context and constructed your own RGT.
3. Now compare your grid to your peers. What is similar? What is different?
4. Now, reflect now upon the data collected from the RGT as similar but different to other data collection methods. Have a conversation in your peer group and discuss aspects of professional learning, for example what events have influenced your learning the most? Who are your role models and why? Why do you learn from some people, but not others? What difference in understanding do these two

approaches (the grid and the conversation) create? Might the RGT help you ask questions and answer them in a unique and exciting way?

	Similarity pole	*1. Your-self in your current role*	*2. Your role model*	*3. Someone else within the professional context*	*Contrast pole*
Construct Pair 1					
Construct Pair 2					
Construct Pair 3					

Conclusion

The examples in the chapter have served to demonstrate that research methods can be exciting and innovative. There are so many ways to determine answers to your questions. Whilst complex in nature, and simplified here for the context, PCT and the RGT are robust and connected research methodologies and data collection methods that can create opportunities for enquiry.

Further reading

Dreyfus, H.L. and Dreyfus, S.E. (1986). *The power of human intuition and expertise in the era of the computer*. New York: Palgrave Macmillan.

Fransella, F., ed. (2003). *International handbook of personal construct psychology*. John Wiley & Sons Ltd.

Fransella, F., Bell, R. and Bannister, D. (2004). *A manual for repertory grid technique*. John Wiley & Sons.

Jankowicz, D. (2004). *The easy guide to repertory grids*. Chichester: John Wiley & Sons Ltd.

Link to the full research study

https://ethos.bl.uk/OrderDetails.do?did=1&uin=uk.bl.ethos.787354

References

Benner, P. (1984). *From novice to expert: Excellence and power in clinical nursing practice*. California: Addison-Wesley Publishing Company.

British Psychological Society. (2019). Code of ethics and conduct. [online] Available at: www.bps.org.uk/news-and-policy/bps-code-ethics-and-conduct.

Brody, D.L. and Hadar, L.L. (2015). Personal professional trajectories of novice and experienced teacher educators in a professional development community. *Teacher Development*, 19(2), pp. 246–266.

Charmaz, K. (2006). *Constructing grounded theory. A practical guide through qualitative analysis*. London: Sage.

Charmaz, K. (2017). The power of constructivist grounded theory for critical inquiry. *Qualitative Inquiry*, 23(1), pp. 34–45.

Darawsheh, W. (2014). Reflexivity in research: Promoting rigour, reliability and validity in qualitative research. *International Journal of Therapy & Rehabilitation*, 21(12), pp. 560–568.

Dreyfus, H.L. and Dreyfus, S.E. (1986). *The power of human intuition and expertise in the era of the computer*. New York: The Free Press.

Eraut, M. (2005). *Expert and expertise: Meanings and perspectives*. Wiley-Blackwell. doi:10.1111/j.1473-6861.2005.00102.x.

Germain, M. and Ruiz, C.E. (2009). Expertise: Myth or reality of a cross-national definition? *Journal of European Industrial Training*, 33(7), pp. 614–634.

Germain, M. and Tejeda, M.J. (2012). A preliminary exploration on the measurement of expertise: An initial development of a psychometric scale. *Human Resource Development Quarterly*, 23(2), pp. 203–232.

Grundtvig Project. (2012). *Handbook of conductive education: Together constructive conductive*. Unpublished manuscript. Available at 2010.

Guba, E.C. (1990). The alternative paradigm dialog. In: E.C. Guba, ed., *The paradigm dialog*. London: Sage, pp. 17.

Hattie, J. (2003). *Distinguishing expert teachers from novice and experienced teachers. Teachers make a difference what is the research evidence?* Paper presented at the Building Teacher Quality, Melbourne, Australia, 19–23 October.

Jankowicz, D. (2004). *The easy guide to repertory grids*. Chichester: John Wiley & Sons Ltd.

Kamath, B.J. and Ashok, H.S. (2015). Religiousness and self-actualization – an empirical study. *Journal of Psychosocial Research*, 10(2), pp. 347–355.

Kelly, G.A. (1963). *A theory of personality: The psychology of personal constructs*. New York: W.W. Norton & Co.

Kinchin, I.M., Cabot, L.B. and Hay, D.B. (2008). Using concept mapping to locate the tacit dimension of clinical expertise: Towards a theoretical framework to support critical reflection on learning. *Learning in Health and Social Care*, 7(2), pp. 93–104.

King, G., Currie, M., Bartlett, D.J., Gilpin, M., Willoughby, C., Tucker, M.A. and Baxter, D. (2007). The development of expertise in pediatric rehabilitation therapists: Changes in approach, self-knowledge, and use of enabling and customizing strategies. *Developmental Neurorehabilitation*, 10(3), pp. 223–240.

Kuipers, K. and Grice, J.W. (2009). Clinical reasoning in neurology: Use of the repertory grid technique to investigate the reasoning of an experienced occupational therapist. [mental map, p282] *Australian Occupational Therapy Journal*, 56(4), pp. 275–284. doi: 10.1111/j.1440-1630.2008.00737.x.

Marsden, D. and Littler, D. (2000). Repertory grid technique – an interpretive research framework. *European Journal of Marketing*, 34(7), pp. 816–834.

McGovern, T.V. and Miller, S.L. (2008). Integrating teacher behaviors with character strengths and virtues for faculty development. *Teaching of Psychology*, 35(4), pp. 278–285. doi: 10.1080/00986280802374609.

Mercer, J. (2007). The challenges of insider research in educational institutions: Wielding a double-edged sword and resolving delicate dilemmas. *Oxford Review of Education*, 33(1), pp. 1–17.

Moore, J. (2012). A personal insight into researcher positionality. *Nurse Researcher*, 19(4), pp. 11–14.

Niemiec, R.M. (2018). *Character strengths interventions*. Boston: Hogrefe.

Pavlovic, J. (2011). Personal construct psychology and social constructionism are not incompatible: Implications of a reframing. *Theory and Psychology*, 21(3), pp. 396–411.

Peterson, C. and Seligman, M.E.P. (2004). *Character strengths and virtues: A handbook and classification*. Oxford: Oxford University Press.

Ralley, C., Allott, R., Hare, D.J. and Wittkowski, A. (2009). The use of the repertory grid technique to examine staff beliefs about clients with dual diagnosis. *Clinical Psychology & Psychotherapy*, 16(2), pp. 148–158.

Raskin, J.D. (2002). Constructivism in psychology: Personal construct psychology, radical constructivism, and social constructionism. In: J.D. Raskin and S.K. Bridges, ed., *Studies in meaning: Exploring constructivist psychology*. New York: Pace University Press, pp. 1–25.

Smith, H.J. (2000). The reliability and validity of structural measures derived from repertory grids. *Journal of Constructivist Psychology*, 13(3), p. 221.

Steed, A. and Mcdonnell, J. (2012). *Experiences with repertory grid analysis for investigating effectiveness of virtual environments* dept. of computer science, University College London, WC1E 6BT @cs.ucl.ac.uk.

Sutcliffe, R., Linfield, R.S. and Geldart, R. (2012). Reflections on the impact on data collection and analysis when 'insiders' carry out research into teacher education. *Research in Education*, 87(1), pp. 104–105.

Szogeczki, L. (2017). *Person-focused rehabilitation: Exploring the psychosocial field of adult conductive education*. Amazon.

Unluer, S. (2012). Being an insider researcher while conducting case study research. *Qualitative Report*, 17.

Wainwright, S.F., Shepard, K.F., Harman, L.B. and Stephens, J. (2011). Factors that influence the clinical decision making of novice and experienced physical therapists. *Physical Therapy*, 91(1), pp. 87–101.

Wink, J. and Wink, D. (2004). *Teaching passionately: What's love got to do with it?* Boston: Pearson.

11 Health and social care inequalities in relation to ethnicity; British South Asian men and nursing careers

Irtiza Qureshi

Introduction

This chapter considers the importance of convergence and intersectionality as part of the research approach for a PhD study which examined the barriers and enablers for British South Asian[1] (BSA) men entering and progressing in the National Health Service (NHS) nursing careers in England.

> **Research question:** What are the barriers and enablers for BSA men entering and progressing in NHS nursing careers in England?

Addressing the shortage of nurses in the NHS is a key government priority. Furthermore, encapsulated in Health Education England's (HEE) widening participation strategy is a focus on diversifying and increasing the number of 'home grown' NHS workforce. Groups such as BSAs (who make up the largest ethnic minority group in England), and men, are underrepresented within the NHS nursing workforce.

DOI: 10.4324/9781003157724-11

Existing evidence highlighted some salient barriers (and enablers) for underrepresented groups entering and progressing in nursing careers. There was however little quantitative or qualitative evidence exploring the experiences of 'home grown' BSA men.

Within this context, the study utilised a convergent parallel mixed methods approach (Johnson and Onwuegbuzie, 2004). The quantitative arm of the study used secondary descriptive data analysis, using proportion ratios and confidence intervals for comparing outcomes between BSA men and British White men (Gardner and Altman, 1986). Secondary descriptive analysis was conducted on national data on applications (*n*=150,445 applicants), acceptances and attrition rates (*n*=416,457 enrolled students) in relation to nursing preregistration courses in England and NHS nursing workforce (*n*=1,254,368 full-time equivalent staff posts) from 2013 to 2016.

The data was retrieved from the relevant databases provided by the relevant agencies, those being, Universities and Colleges Application Service (UCAS) for applications and acceptances to nursing courses, Higher Education Statistics Agency (HESA) for attrition from nursing courses and HEE for NHS workforce data.

The qualitative arm of the study used focus group discussions (Creswell, 2018) with BSA young men and BSA parents and carers in Luton to explore their views on barriers and enablers for BSA men choosing nursing education and careers (*n*=22 young men, 35 parents).

In addition, one-to-one interviews (Bowling, 2009) were conducted nationally with professionals and stakeholders (*n*=5 nurses, 5 other professionals) to ascertain their views on the subject. Participants were recruited purposively, deploying snowballing techniques where appropriate (Rajacich et al., 2013).

Critically, the study was underpinned by an intersectional conceptual framework (Crenshaw, 1991). Intersectionality added value to this study because it helped consider the specific experience of BSA men in this context. This had never been done for this group and therefore the use of intersectionality made this a unique feature of this study – both adding value to results and findings and developing the use of intersectionality as a concept in health service research.

Key converged results and findings incorporating an intersectional approach

- Unconscious bias in nursing education institutional practice may be a barrier to BSA men entering nursing education.
- There is a 'glass ceiling' in place for BSA male nurses' career progression and this may be part of institutional racism acting as a barrier.
- Male relatives' views were a barrier for BSA men entering into nursing careers.
- BSA men suggested aspects of BSA masculinities were seen as enablers for BSA men entering into nursing careers.

Converging results and findings and applying an intersectional analysis

Now that we know the context of the study, what it set out to do and what the results and findings were, we can start to consider some aspects of how the study was done. In particular, we will focus on how the results and findings of the study were analysed. Remember this was a mixed methods study which converged its quantitative results and qualitative findings. Alongside this, the study was underpinned by an intersectional conceptual framework. We will now consider what convergence and intersectionalism are before considering how they were applied in this study.

Convergence

One of the benefits of using a mixed methods approach is that a researcher can triangulate results and findings (Greene, Caracelli and Graham, 1989). One aim of triangulation is to determine whether the results/findings from different analyses within a piece of research 'converge' or 'tell the same story'; if they do, then they are more dependable; therefore, we can assign more validity to these results/

findings (Denzin and Lincoln, 1994). If the results/findings tell slightly different stories, then we can conclude that there is partial convergence. If they tell completely different stories, then we can conclude there is dissonance. The term dissonance means that the two sets of data are at odds. This itself can be useful as dissonant findings can be utilised as a starting place for a new or more nuanced understanding of a phenomenon (Miles, Huberman and Saldaña, 2014). As useful as this process of converging results and findings is, unfortunately there are few examples of how to implement this process (Farmer et al., 2006). Therefore, we will use this study to explore what the process is and how it can add value to a piece of research.

Intersectionalism

Health service researchers have previously used a number of theoretical approaches to analysing the disadvantage faced by minority groups. These approaches have included critical race theory (Ackerman-Barger and Hummel, 2015); everyday racism (Mapedzahama et al., 2012); gender-based analysis (Choiniere, MacDonnell and Shamonda, 2010); unconscious bias (Williamson, 2018) and microaggressions (Solorzano, Ceja and Yosso, 2000) amongst others. However, a range of studies (Bagilhole, 2010; Viruell-Fuentes, Miranda and Abdulrahim, 2012) argue for the use of an intersectionalist lens on existing policies. They argue that policy development has for too long been focussed on singular constructs in identity formation, leaving those involved with 'lens fatigue' having to constantly reassess levels of inequality across singular groupings such as men and women in gender bias. Intersectionalism was developed by Kimberle Crenshaw in order to analyse the position of ethnic minority women in the United States. Intersectionality acknowledges that multiple factors have an influence on any phenomenon including ethnicity, faith and gender at individual level and power dynamics at a more structural and systemic level (Crenshaw, 1991).

Now that we have a shared understanding of the terms, we can see how they were applied in this study. Remember, this study aimed to answer the following research question:

Research question: What are the barriers and enablers for the BSA men entering and progressing in NHS nursing careers in England?

In order to answer the question, this study gathered quantitative results (a review of applications to nursing preregistration courses and NHS nursing workforce data) as well as qualitative findings (BSA community and professional stakeholder views on the barriers and enablers for BSA men entering and progressing in nursing careers). Converging these results and findings allows us to analyse the data and make meta-inferences which go beyond single method analysis (Onwuegbuzie et al., 2009). This study adapted a model of convergence based on a six-step protocol. The protocol was developed specifically for health research (Farmer et al., 2006).

The six steps in the Farmer et al. (2006) protocol consist of:

1. *Sorting* – The findings related to the research question from each data set are sorted and separated from the rest of the data into two files. Contents of both files are reviewed to identify the key themes discussed in each data set to create a unified list of themes to compare for presence and frequency, meaning and examples. These themes form the rows of a convergence coding matrix used to summarise similarities and differences between the two sets of results/findings.
2. *Convergence coding* – A convergence coding scheme is devised to help determine convergence or dissonance between the two sets of results/findings. The data convergence codes included agreement (AG); partial agreement (PA); silence (S) and dissonance (DA).
3. *Convergence assessment* – Next, we assess the results/findings and implement the convergence coding scheme.
4. *Completeness comparison* – Then the two sets of results/findings are compared to highlight both similar and unique contributions to the research question, ultimately creating a summary of the unified findings of the two sets of results/findings. This is done based on the

principle that each data set on its own provides part of the story for this research question, but together, they contribute to a higher level of analysis and a broader understanding of the research question.

5. *Researcher comparison* – This is when multiple relevant researchers (if appropriate) come to an agreement between themselves on whether their results/findings have been correctly assessed and coded.
6. Feedback – The final step in this process is sharing the results of the convergence exercise with a wider research team and wider stakeholders such as research participants (if appropriate) for feedback/comment.

The relevance of converged results and findings will now be discussed in the context of an intersectional analysis. Application of the intersectional approach provides a useful conceptual framework to understand BSA men's experience of nursing through the lens of intersecting factors such as ethnicity and gender. By converging, analysing and discussing the results and findings with an emphasis on these intersecting factors, the similarities and differences between BSA men and other men become more apparent. This adds to the deeper understanding of the overall perception, experience and choices of BSA men and nursing. We will consider this analysis using the identified barriers for BSA men entering and progressing into nursing as they emerged as findings within the study.

Barrier 1 Lack of knowledge and awareness or unconscious bias within nursing education institutions as a barrier

Although one of the themes emerging as a barrier suggested a lack of knowledge and awareness of the nursing profession on the part of BSA men (and the BSA community), quantitative results showed that they were twice as likely to apply for nursing preregistration courses as their British White male counterparts. This demonstrates dissonance when converging the results and findings, as the higher application rate could suggest that BSA men are more aware of nursing education and careers than their White male counterparts. One explanation for why they are less likely to be accepted may be

Table 11.1 Converged results and findings in relation to lack of knowledge and awareness and application rates

Theme/ sub-themes	*Quantitative results*	*Young people's findings*	*Parents' findings*	*Nurse findings*
Lack of knowledge and awareness (including lack of careers information).	BSA men twice as likely to apply for nursing courses.	Many young people said they did not receive a great deal of information on nursing as a career at school or college.	Many parents said they had never even considered nursing as a career for their sons.	Nurses generally acknowledged that nursing was not even considered as a career option for young BSA men.

to do with unconscious bias in the selection processes and practice within nursing education institutions (Bhopal, 2017; Arday and Mirza, 2018). This rationale may be further consolidated when considering results showed that BSA men were half as likely to be accepted onto nursing preregistration courses. Furthermore, they were 18% more likely to leave their courses without the intended award in comparison to their White male counterparts (see Table 11.1).

This converged set of results and findings highlight a specific experience for BSA men due to their ethnicity and gender in the nursing profession. Intersectionalism provides a particular perspective on analysing the context of BSA men in nursing considering both their ethnicity and their gender in the nursing profession. The evidence base would suggest that unconscious bias could be a barrier in this experience for BSA men entering the nursing profession (Solorzano, Ceja and Yosso, 2000; Cornish and Jones, 2013; Sporek, 2015); however, this issue requires further research.

Barrier 2 Pay and conditions as a barrier (including a glass ceiling and institutional racism)

Critically, the results from this research suggest that BSA male nurses do not enjoy the benefits of comparatively higher pay and more prestigious roles through their patriarchal advantage in the nursing profession. This is especially significant when considering

Table 11.2 Converged results and findings in relation to pay and conditions

Theme/ sub-themes	*Quantitative results*	*Young people's findings*	*Parents' findings*	*Nurse findings*
Pay and conditions	Lack of senior roles 3.1% for BSA men compared to 9.4% for white men.	Many young people did not perceive nursing as financially rewarding.	Many parents did not perceive nursing as financially rewarding.	Some nurses suggested there was a glass ceiling in place for them.
Pay and conditions	Over-representation of BSA men in Adult, Emergency and General Nursing (by 40%).	Many young people felt there was a lot of responsibility and long shift hours.	Many parents felt it was not respected and valued as a profession.	Some nurses suggested the level of pay was not commensurate with the role (especially in the south east of the country).

the intersectional nature of this study. With regard to converging the results and findings, this showed agreement across all objectives, as demonstrated in Table 11.2.

The evidence base would suggest that BSA men would face a barrier to their career progression due to their ethnicity by way of institutional racism (Allan et al., 2004; Qureshi, Ali and Randhawa, 2020). However, this barrier could be offset for BSA men by virtue of their gender and therefore enjoying a patriarchal dividend in the nursing profession (Herdman and Badir, 2008). The results from this review suggest that the patriarchal dividend does not apply to BSA men, and therefore their gender does not supersede their ethnicity in this context. The results of this study show that like their female BAME counterparts (Brathwaite, 2018), BSA men are less likely to hold senior or management positions than their white counterparts.

Barrier 3 Male relatives' views as a barrier

Converging the results of findings from focus groups and interviews demonstrated partial agreement across participant views, as

Table 11.3 Converged findings in relation to family views

Theme/ sub-themes	*Quantitative results*	*Young people's findings*	*Parents' findings*	*Nurse findings*
Family views	N/A	Young people generally reported parental views as a barrier, as they felt their parents would not consider nursing as a suitable occupation for them.	Fathers did not consider nursing as a viable career option for their sons. Mothers were more open to this idea.	Some of the nurses reported a negative response from their male family/friends when deciding to enter the nursing profession.

both BSA parents and BSA male nurses agreed that family views (especially male relatives' views) were a barrier (see Table 11.3).

BSA male nurses also reported the men in their families felt particularly strongly against them being a nurse. Conversely, some talked of the female members in their family being initially (and consistently) supportive of them wanting to go into nursing. Findings from focus groups also indicated BSA mothers being more open to their sons being nurses, especially when considering known BSA male nurse role models. These findings point to a difference in family views as a barrier for BSA people and nursing. The views of fathers, brothers and other male relatives within BSA families may be a stronger deterrent for BSA men entering nursing than their female relatives' views. If this is the case, this finding adds to the body of knowledge on the subject.

Barrier 4 British South Asian masculinities; barrier or enabler?

The converged findings show dissonance across participant views of BSA masculinities, as some saw BSA masculinities as a barrier whilst others saw it as an enabler (see Table 11.4).

These findings are even more interesting when considered within an intersectional context. For example, even though the South Asian community identifying certain aspects of South Asian masculinity being compatible with qualities required of nurses is interesting on its own. However, when further analysed it becomes clear that it is particularly BSA men (young men and fathers) found this to be true.

Table 11.4 Converged findings in relation to BSA masculinities

Theme/ sub-themes	*Quantitative results*	*Young people's findings*	*Parents' findings*	*Nurse findings*
Barrier				
Masculinity and gender	N/A	Many young people saw nursing as a female profession.	Many parents saw nursing as a female profession.	Nurses generally acknowledged the public perception of nursing as a feminised profession and felt this was a barrier for young men.
Enabler				
Masculinity	N/A	In some instances, young people found that key qualities required for nursing were compatible with key characteristics of South Asian masculinity.	Many fathers found that key qualities required for nursing were compatible with key characteristics of South Asian masculinity. Mothers were not in agreement to the same extent as fathers were.	Some nurses felt that the expected attitudes and behaviours within South Asian masculinities did not align with key qualities required of nursing professionals – yet, some nurses felt that there was alignment and that it could be an enabler.

Far fewer women (mothers) espoused this view. Therefore, using an intersectional approach we can see that there is a difference in the perceptions of the two different genders within the BSA ethnic group in relation to masculinity and the nursing profession. Gender seemed to be the defining intersecting factor on the perceptions of the nursing profession within the context of ethnicity.

An intersectional analysis of the findings from one-to-one interviews and the existing evidence base does highlight the difference in perceptions of BSA male and female nurses. Within the evidence base (Daly, Swindlehurst and Johal, 2003) female BSA nurses did not report any perceived racism or discrimination in their nursing education or career. However, the majority of BSA male nurses interviewed in this study did report perceived discrimination as a career/pay limiting phenomenon in nursing. As such, gender seems to be a differential factor in the experience or perceived experience of people of the same ethnicity within the nursing profession in this case.

Reviewing research challenges and lessons learnt

One of the practical challenges for health service researchers when investigating the circumstance of ethnic minorities is navigating the differing approaches to ethnic categorisation. This was a clear problem for this particular study.

This research used various data sources to build a picture of the quantitative context. Although the national census ethnic grouping categories are widely used for benchmarking purposes, it may be that categorisation systems differ in their approach to ethnic grouping across the nursing system (i.e. across nursing education institutions and nursing profession organisations). These organisations include universities, Universities and Colleges Admissions Service (UCAS), Higher Education Statistics Agency (HESA), NHS employer organisations such as Trusts, HEE and the Nursing and Midwifery Council (NMC).

The quantitative data gathering exercise for this study demonstrated some of the inconsistencies in how data was collected, grouped and disseminated. For example, although both UCAS and HESA used similar ethnic group categorisations (based on the 18 census groups) for data capture, upon request, UCAS provided ethnic data based on 14 ethnic groupings. However, HESA provided only derived ethnicity grouping breakdowns into ten groups (collapsing all 'mixed' ethnicities into the 'other' category). UCAS also rounded down data to the nearest five. HESA did not do this. All justifications for limitations placed on data dissemination were in relation to data protection. The end result of these inconsistencies was that it was challenging to compare like with like within this study, and therefore it is one of the study limitations.

Regarding the nursing workforce data, there is a more general problem that the male proportion of the NHS nursing workforce is so low that any further analysis within the male cohort becomes even more disproportional to the overall workforce. BAME men representation varies across different ethnic groups and also masks the nursing specialism that certain ethnic groups are working in. The Asian/Asian British categorisation of ethnicity does not provide the detail of how many of the categorised cohort are defining themselves as BSA, in other words, of South Asian ethnic descent but educated in the UK/'home grown' nurses. This set of statistics represents a number of overseas staff who may class themselves as Asian/Asian British, and therefore this represents not only a problem in data categorisation but also indicates the long-standing issue of reliance on overseas recruitment to nursing positions in the NHS. The widening participation agenda is specifically aimed at developing a 'home grown' (Malhotra, 2006; Ali et al., 2018; Munn, 2018) healthcare workforce. This initial consideration of data gathering showed that the current categorisation systems do not provide clarity in seeking to understand the true picture of who is 'home grown' and genuinely BSA, and therefore problematic for the widening participation agenda.

Remember, a major issue this categorisation system presented was that it made it difficult to identify the number of 'home grown' BSA people in the workforce. It is important to define what is meant by 'home grown' in this context. For the purposes of this research, 'home grown' refers to those of South Asian ethnic descent but educated or trained in the UK. Although the key criteria here are ethnicity and geographical location of education, it is relevant to consider socialisation for South Asian immigrant and minority ethnic groups, as it is an important variable in their understanding of their values, beliefs, culture and identity (Inman et al., 2007; Tummala-Narra, Inman and Ettigi, 2011; Daga and Raval, 2018).

Certain assumptions had to be made in this study about who may qualify as BSA. This study has set out the criteria of being of South Asian descent and educated in the UK as key to qualifying as the target population. However, as ethnic identity is subjective, data is subject to self-identification (in the case of the national census for example). In fact, some researchers would question the value of using a concept such as ethnicity in health research at all (Simpson, 2000; Cho, 2006). Some countries do not record ethnicity as part of their census (Hickman, 2011); there is no one unequivocal definition of ethnicity (Nazroo, 1998; Chaturvedi, 2001). All researchers must be alert to the complexity of how groups self-identify and self-report their ethnicity.

Activity 1

Imagine you are researching particular health outcomes for a particular ethnic minority group. Write a 200-word abstract setting out your research proposal.

You will need to:

- Decide what the ethnic group is.
- Decide what the outcomes are (e.g. analysing Body Mass Index).
- Write down how you will go about defining your target population.
- Write down how you will compare the health outcomes (e.g. using proportional ratios to compare between ethnic groups).
- Write down how you will collect your data.

How research relates to policy and practice

As explained earlier, identifying 'home grown' BSA people was a challenge. Furthermore, we can identify 'home grown' nursing students because the UCAS system allows for the segregation of 'domestic' applications/acceptances. However, this is not the case for NHS Trusts.

This study made it apparent that many of those working within nursing and equalities do know of BSA male nurses but that they are not 'home grown' nurses. This could indicate that the vast majority of those BSA male nurses on NHS Electronic Service Register (even with British nationality) are not 'home grown'. They have no other choice than indicating they are Asian/Asian British and then either Indian, Pakistani, Bangladeshi or other – thus conflating 'home grown' with internationally trained/recruited nurses. Therefore, we cannot identify where the destinations for 'home grown' BSA nurse students are in the workforce. These questions lead to the fundamental challenge of how we can have policies to develop a 'home grown' workforce if we don't know who they are and where they are.

Activity 2

- The results and findings from this research have been disseminated through peer-reviewed academic journals.
- How else could this research be disseminated to better inform policy and practice?

Ethical issues

With regard to the quantitative data, certain ethical implications concerning data protection of individual applicants had to be taken into consideration. The small numbers of applications from some ethnic groups and data confidentiality policy meant that UCAS cohort data was only made available rounded to the nearest five.

With regard to the qualitative data, all data collected were anonymised, and no personal or individually identifiable information was shared. Consent forms explaining all participatory implications were used as well as participant information sheets. The data-gathering process was further reviewed in order to assure compliance with recent national General Data Protection Regulation (GDPR) guidance. Formal ethical approval was also obtained from the University of Bedfordshire.

Key learning

- Converging results and findings can strengthen validity of your research.
- Using an intersectional approach can provide a more sophisticated analysis of the experience of marginalised subjects.
- Ethnicity is a contested and complex concept.
- Identifying a target population can be more difficult than we might think!

Note

1 The term British South Asian refers to those people of South Asian ethnicity, born and or socialised in the UK (Ali, Kalra and Sayyid, 2006). It is most closely aligned with the ethnic group definition used in the 2011 census (Office of National Statistics, 2011) where Asian/Asian British refers to Pakistani, Indian and Bangladeshi (not including Chinese or any other Asian background).

Further reading

Bartley, M. (2004). *Health inequality: An introduction to theories, concepts, and methods*. Cambridge, UK: Polity Press.

Qureshi, I., Ali, N. and Randhawa, G. (2020). British South Asian male nurses' views on the barriers and enablers to entering and progressing in nursing careers. *Journal of Nursing Management*, 28, 892–902. https://doi.org/10.1111/jonm.13017.

References

Ali, N., Kalra, V.S. and Sayyid, S. (2006). *A postcolonial people: South Asians in Britain*. Edited by N. Ali and Salman Sayyid. London: C. Hurst and Co.

Ali, N., et al. (2018). Barriers and enablers for UK "home grown" south Asian prospective students choosing nursing and midwifery courses and careers. *Diversity and Equality in Health and Care*, 15(4), pp. 190–197.

Ackerman-Barger, K. and Hummel, F. (2015) 'Critical race Theory as a lens for Exploring inclusion and Equity in Nursing Education', The Journal of Theory Construction & Testing, 19(2), pp. 39–46.

Allan, H.T., et al. (2004). The social reproduction of institutional racism: Internationally recruited nurses' experiences of the British health services. *Diversity in Health & Social Care*, 1(2), pp. 117–125.

Arday, J. and Mirza, H.S. (2018). *Dismantling race in higher education: Racism, whiteness and decolonizing the academy*. London: Palgrave Macmillan. doi: 10.1007/978-3-319-60261-5.

Bagilhole, B. (2010). Applying the lens of intersectionality to UK equal opportunities and diversity policies. *Canadian Journal of Administrative Sciences*, 27(3), pp. 263–271. doi: 10.1002/cjas.167.

Bhopal, K. (2017). Addressing racial inequalities in higher education: Equity, inclusion and social justice. *Ethnic and Racial Studies*, 40(13), pp. 2293–2299. doi: 10.1080/01419870.2017.1344267.

Bowling, A. (2009). *Research methods in health*, 3rd ed. New York: Open University.

Brathwaite, B. (2018). Black, Asian and minority ethnic female nurses: Colonialism, power and racism. *British Journal of Nursing*, 27(5), pp. 254–258. doi: 10.12968/bjon.2018.27.5.254.

Chaturvedi, N. (2001). Ethnicity as an epidemiological determinant – Crudely racist or crucially important? *International Journal of Epidemiology*, 30, pp. 925–927. doi: 10.1093/ije/30.5.925.

Cho, M.K. (2006). Racial and ethnic categories in biomedical research: There is no baby in the bathwater. *Journal of Law Medicine and Ethics*, 34(3).

Choiniere, J.A., MacDonnell, J. and Shamonda, H. (2010). Walking the talk: Insights into dynamics of race and gender for nurses. *Policy, Politics, and Nursing Practice*, 11(4), pp. 317–325. doi: 10.1177/1527154410396222.

Cornish, T. and Jones, P. (2013). *Unconscious bias and higher education*. London: Equality Challenge Unit.

Crenshaw, K. (1991). Mapping the margins: Intersectionality, identity politics, and violence against women of color. *Stanford Law Review*, 43(6), pp. 1241–1299. doi: 10.2307/1229039.

Creswell, J.W. (2018). *Research design: Qualitative, quantitative and mixed methods approaches*, 5th ed. London: Sage Publications. doi: 10.3109/08941939.2012.723954.

Daga, S.S. and Raval, V.V. (2018). Ethnic-racial socialization, model minority experience, and psychological functioning among south Asian American emerging adults: A preliminary mixed-methods study. *Asian American Journal of Psychology*, 9(1), pp. 17–31. doi: 10.1037/aap0000108.

Daly, W., Swindlehurst, L. and Johal, P. (2003). Exploration into the recruitment of South Asian nurses. *British Journal of Nursing*, 12(11). [online] Available at: www.statistics.gov.uk/census.

Denzin, N.K. and Lincoln, Y.S. (1994). *Handbook of qualitative research*. Sage. Available at: www.uncg.edu/hdf/facultystaff/Tudge/Guba%20&%20Lincoln%201994.pdf.

Farmer, T., et al. (2006). Developing and implementing a triangulation protocol for qualitative health research. *Qualitative Health Research*, 16(3), pp. 377–394. doi: 10.1177/1049732305285708.

Gardner, M.J. and Altman, D.G. (1986). Statistics in medicine confidence intervals rather than P values: Estimation rather than hypothesis testing. *British Medical Journal (Clinical research ed.)*, 292(6522), pp. 746–750. doi: 10.1136/bmj.292.6522.746.

Greene, J.C., Caracelli, V.J. and Graham, W.F. (1989). Toward a conceptual framework for mixed-method evaluation designs. *Educational Evaluation and Policy Analysis*, 11(3), pp. 255–274. doi: 10.3102/01623737011003255.

Herdman, E. and Badir, A. (2008). Gender equality or patriarchal dividend: Structural change in Turkish nursing. *Nursing and Health Sciences*, 10(2), pp. 159–163. doi: 10.1111/j.1442-2018.2008.00384.x.

Hickman, M.J. (2011). Census ethnic categories and second-generation identities: A study of the Irish in England and Wales. *Journal of Ethnic and Migration Studies*, 37(1), pp. 79–97. doi: 10.1080/1369183X.2011.523005.

Inman, A.G., et al. (2007). Cultural transmission: Influence of contextual factors in Asian Indian immigrant parents' experiences. *Journal of Counseling Psychology*, 54(1), pp. 93–100. doi: 10.1037/0022-0167.54.1.93.

Johnson, R.B. and Onwuegbuzie, A.J. (2004). Mixed methods research: A research paradigm whose time has come. *Educational Research*, 33(14), pp. 14–26.

Malhotra, G. (2006). *Grow your own : Creating the condition for sustainable workforce development*. King's Fund.

Mapedzahama, V. et al. (2012). Black nurse in white space? Rethinking the in/visibility of race within the Australian nursing workplace. *Nursing Inquiry*, 19(2), pp. 153–164. doi: 10.1111/j.1440-1800.2011.00556.x.

Miles, M.B., Huberman, A.M. and Saldaña, J. (2014). *Qualitative data analysis*, 3rd ed. Arizona: Sage.

Munn, F. (2018). Why nurturing homegrown talent is best for every nation. *Nursing Standard*, 32(20).

Nazroo, J.Y. (1998). Genetic, cultural or socio-economic vulnerability? Explaining ethnic inequalities in health. *Sociology of Health & Illness*, 20(5), pp. 710–730.

Onwuegbuzie, A.J., et al. (2009). Mixed data analysis : Advanced integration techniques. *International Journal of Mul*, 3(1), pp. 13–33.

Qureshi, I., Ali, N. and Randhawa, G. (2020). British South Asian male nurses' views on the barriers and enablers to entering and progressing in nursing careers. *Journal of Nursing Management*, 28(4), pp. 892–902. doi: 10.1111/jonm.13017.

Rajacich, D., et al. (2013). If they do call you a nurse, it is always a "male nurse": Experiences of men in the nursing profession. *Nursing Forum*, 48(1).

Simpson, B. (2000). Imagined genetic communities. *Anthropology Today*, 16(3), pp. 3–6. doi: 10.1111/1467-8322.00023.

Solorzano, D., Ceja, M. and Yosso, T. (2000). Critical race theory, racial microaggressions, and campus racial climate: The experiences of African American college students. *The Journal of Negro Education*, 69(1 & 2), pp. 60–73. doi: 10.1080/095183998236926.

Sporek, P. (2015). Unconscious bias. *British Journal of Midwifery*, 23(12), p. 910. doi: 10.1126/science.1219009.Equality.

Tummala-Narra, P., Inman, A.G. and Ettigi, S.P. (2011). Asian Indians' responses to discrimination: A mixed-method examination of identity, coping, and self-esteem. *Asian American Journal of Psychology*, 2(3), pp. 205–218. doi: 10.1037/a0025555.

Viruell-Fuentes, E.A., Miranda, P.Y. and Abdulrahim, S. (2012). More than culture: Structural racism, intersectionality theory, and immigrant health. *Social Science and Medicine*, 75(12), pp. 2099–2106. doi: 10.1016/j.socscimed.2011.12.037.

Williamson, S. (2018). Unconscious Bias Training: The "Silver Bullet" for Gender Equity ? *Australian Journal of Public Administration*, 77(3), pp. 355–359. doi: 10.1111/1467-8500.12313.

Index

Note: Locators in *italic* and **bold** refer to figures and tables respectively, and locators followed by "n" refer to end notes.

For Product Safety Concerns and Information please contact our EU representative GPSR@taylorandfrancis.com Taylor & Francis Verlag GmbH, Kaufingerstraße 24, 80331 München, Germany